MW00881307

Intermittent fasting for women

Definitive and Complete Guide to Fasting

Everything You Need to Know about Being Successful at Fasting

RACHELE PARKESSON

1

2

Table of Contents

Introduction

This book contains all the essential information you need to know about fasting.

Simply put, fasting means not eating any food for a given period of time. It appears like anybody could do it on their own without having to refer to medical experts or even a guidebook. Intermittent fasting losing weight is among the most efficient ways to shed additional pounds. The ideas about the intermittent rapid loss of weight challenge most of the previous beliefs on this subject. Those who want new ways to lose weight quickly embraced their ideas effectively. However, fasting is not as easy as it sounds.

There are several nuances to it that can spell the difference between a successful fast and a failed attempt. Even the tiniest tweaks to your fasting plan can enhance or diminish the benefits that you could get from a fast.

In this book, you will learn about:
- whether or not you can benefit from fasting;
- the positive effects of fasting on your health;
- the highlights of the history of fasting;
- the right fasting method for you;
- what to expect once you have begun fasting;

- the factors that affect the weight loss effects of fasting;
- the proper way to track your progress while fasting;
- the methods to ward off the potential negative effects of fasting;
- an effective and detailed kick-start fasting plan;
- recipes of suggested dishes that you can eat while fasting; and
- examples of simple exercises that you can do to enhance the positive effects of fasting on your health.

This book aims to guide in discovering the best fasting method for you, as well as ease you into the process of abstaining from food in a healthy manner. Fasting can be quite challenging, but with commitment and discipline, you can be sure that the rewards would be great.

Thanks for downloading this book, I hope you enjoy it!

Rachele

Chapter 1 – Determining Who Can Benefit from Fasting

Intermittent fasting is not a diet. You may be tired of trying anything with the word "diet" in it when it comes to losing those extra pounds. Intermittent Fasting is a way to lose weight that involves a structured program of when you should eat and when you should not eat. You will be able to create your own plan that will suit your needs, especially if you can go through with it quickly for a whole day! Quick means spending twelve full hours empty before a meal. You can increase your fasting time later when the program continues.

If you have been attempting to lose weight, you probably have tried diets like the Atkins diet which is based on the frequent eating theory. Those who advocate such diets advise you to eat often throughout the day. The idea behind those food plans is to make your metabolism work faster only by eating more. The quicker your metabolism, the faster you will lose weight. However, the more food you ate, the more you wished to eat, and the more your weight was left intact. If you decide to enroll in an intermittent program, your meal frequency will have to be reduced. You will have to do without breakfast sometimes.

You probably sleep 6 to 8 hours. Your body is in fasting mode during this time. When your body is fasting, it generates more insulin. More insulin in your body increases your sensitivity to insulin. If your organism is more sensitive to insulin, you lose more fat. The brilliance of the intermittent weight loss program is that you spend your breakfast on extending the insulin sensitivity of your body. This means that your body will be losing fat for a long time which translates into losing more weight.

A more extended fasting mode also has a great effect on your body's hormone levels. Your body produces growth hormones by skipping breakfast or eating at a specific time. Producing growth hormone is essential when you are trying to lose weight because it helps your body to do this exact task. If your weight loss program is intermittent, your growth hormone levels are usually at their highest which results in losing more weight. High levels of growth hormone also have several other health benefits in your body. This program is just excellent!

Fasting is highly recommended for anyone who wishes to live a longer and healthier life. Many medical experts also recognize this as an excellent way to manage and reverse several chronic health conditions, such as heart diseases and cancer. However, studies show that fasting may not be effective for all types of people.

As with any major health decision that you have to make, it is best to seek first the professional opinion of your physician before committing yourself to significant changes in your lifestyle and diet. Fasting may aggravate any existing health condition, especially the ones that you may not be aware of at this point.

Have an open discussion with your doctor about your goals for fasting, as well as the probable side-effects this activity could have on your health. By doing so, you would be able to engage in fasting without any serious reservations about your wellbeing.

For your reference, here is a rundown of specific groups of people, and their respective likelihood of benefiting from fasting:

- Children

    Average children, up to the age of 18, are not recommended to fast. At most, health experts may advise parents to control the frequency of their child's meals throughout the day. Children should not be abstaining from food for long periods of time. The nutrition they gain from their meals are essential for their growth and development.

Even overweight children are not exempted from this. Parents, with the guidance of the child's pediatrician or a nutritionist, should try restructuring first the child's diet. The objective for such a move is to prevent the child from consuming junk food and too much sugar, and replace them with healthier options.

Once the overweight child begins eating a well-balanced diet, most parents do not have any reason left to wonder if child has to go through a fast to lose the excess weight.

If you still think that a child below the age of 18 would benefit from a fast, you should consult with the child's physician first.

- Healthy Adults

    Being in good health does not exclude healthy adults from benefiting from fasting. In fact, going into a fast from time to time may be helpful in sustaining their current health condition.

- High-Level Athletes

    Several benefits of fasting are attractive for many athletes. Fasting enables the body to recover faster from being strained, and it improves the absorption of nutrients of the digestive system. Both benefits are critical in the process of developing muscles and increasing physical strength.

Athletes should take extra care when adapting fasting into their normal routines. Experts do not suggest going on a fast right before and during game days. Fasting should not also be done when the athlete has to engage in intense and extended practice sessions. Doing any of these would seriously deplete them to the point that the continual act of abstaining from food becomes harmful to their health.

- Pregnant Women

  Multiple studies have been conducted on the effects of fasting among pregnant Muslim women during Ramadan. To date, researchers have found that fasting has no negative effects on the mother or the child.

  Pregnancy, however, is a highly sensitive state, so pregnant women are encouraged to get the approval of their respective doctors first before entering a fast.

- Vegetarians or Vegans

  Fasting is compatible with almost every type of lifestyle or diet. Due to the dietary restrictions of vegetarians and vegans, the effects of fasting may even be enhanced when implemented properly.

- Individuals with Type-2 Diabetes

  Fasting has long been used by medical experts as a method of reversing Type-2 Diabetes. Various research studies on this strategy show consistent results indicating the positive effects of fasting to diabetic people. Still, if you are diabetic too, you should consult first with your doctor before adapting any form of fasting.

- Individuals who are Immunosuppressed

  People who are suffering from HIV, AIDS, lupus, different types of cancer, or any similar disorders related to the immune system should seek the opinion of their physicians before making any major lifestyle or dietary changes, such as fasting.

  Though fasting is largely beneficial to most people, it may wreak havoc to the delicate balance of bodily chemicals and processes of an immunosuppressed individual.

- Individuals with Eating Disorders

  An eating disorder is rooted upon the physical, mental, and emotional aspects of a person suffering from it. Therefore, there is no guarantee that fasting may help resolve these food-related issues. Those who have been diagnosed with eating disorders should get the approval of their psychotherapists first before applying the principles of fasting into their lives.

As you can see, almost every group of people may benefit from fasting. However, most groups are also encouraged to get the opinion of medical experts prior to making a commitment to fasting.

In case you want to do a preliminary self-assessment before your consultation, here is a set of guide questions that you may reflect upon to determine whether or not fasting is for you.

- How well do handle hunger pangs?
- Can you fully commit to fasting for at least three months?
- Do you think you have the physical and mental fortitude to last through an entire fasting period?

- How would you describe your current diet?
- How would you describe your current lifestyle?
- How do you regard the thought of having to exercise regularly?
- Do you have support system who can motivate you and hold you accountable while you are fasting?

It is best if you would write down your answers to these questions in a personal journal. Refer to your responses before making a final decision regarding fasting. Even if your physician has given you clearance to pursue with this, you must be willing to commit yourself, and go through the highs and lows of fasting as best you can.

Take the time to reflect upon the questions given above. Doing so would help you figure out if you have what it takes to reap the numerous benefits of fasting.

It is also worth mentioning the groups of people that shouldn't fast intermittently:

• Women who are pregnant or breastfeeding, unless they are allowed to do so by their doctors.

• Those who are underweight and malnourished.

• Children under 18 and elders.

• Those with gout.

• Those that have Gastroesophageal reflux (GERD) disease.

• Those with eating disorders should consult their physicians first.

• Diabetes and insulin patients must contact their physicians in advance, as dosages must be through.

• The drug consumers must consult their physicians first as the timing of medicines may be affected.

• Those with high stress or cortisol issues should not be rapid since fasting is another stressor.

• Those who train very hard most days of the week.

Chapter 2 – Why Fasting Is Good for Health

While fasting has existed for thousands of years, the advantages of intermittent fasting for fat loss have only recently been investigated. The intermittent weight loss program differs radically from those promoted on the market for most weight loss programs. However, when it comes to weight loss, her ideas are scientifically sound. If you're serious about weight loss, you should give this program a go. When done properly, fasting can make you feel better and look better. To prove this point, here are the various positive effects of fasting on your body and mind.

- Abstaining from food enables the body to burn more fat.

  In most cases, fasting is considered as one of the safest means to lose weight. It initiates lipolysis, or the process of unlocking stored fats and releasing them into the bloodstream as a source of energy for the body.

  After your body has completely digested the last meal you had before entering a fast, lipolysis takes over to sustain your energy levels. Studies show that this usually takes place within the first two hours of a fast.

However, releasing the fatty acids into your bloodstream is not enough to ensure weight loss. When you eat too soon after their release, the body would store them back through a process called re-esterification. Therefore, to prevent this from occurring, you must sustain your fast for various periods of time. This would allow the oxidation, or the fat-burning process, to take place.

You may further augment this by exercising while you are in a fast. Doing so would ensure that none of the released fatty acids would remain in your body as stored fats.

- Fasting, coupled with the right exercise routines, can help you gain muscle faster.

A special protein in the human body called mammalian target of rapamycin (mTOR) is primarily responsible for the development of muscle. It must, however, be regulated because too much or too little of it can have adverse effects on the body. For instance, when you go over the ideal mTOR activity for extended periods of time, it will increase your risk of irregular cell growth. This could then lead to the onset of various forms of cancer.

Fasting is one of the most effective means of controlling mTOR activities within your body. To understand how, you must learn how mTOR is activated first.

○ Through the release of insulin hormones into your bloodstream

Insulin is responsible for regulating your blood sugar. It is also essential for transporting nutrients into cells.

Insulin is released by the pancreas whenever you eat. However, chronic insulin elevation is linked to serious health conditions, such as diabetes, Alzheimer's disease, and heart diseases.

○ Through intense exercises

Engaging in intense exercises initially suppresses mTOR activities. By the time you have ended your routine, in a significant amount of potential for muscle development would have accumulated in the mTOR. This will be released like a coiled spring once you have consumed food after exercising.

Fasting helps in regulating mTOR because it can restore the balance in your insulin levels. Furthermore, the more you are able to sustain it at those levels, the more sensitive you become to the effects of insulin to your body. Over time, you would only need less insulin in order to perform as you would normally do.

Exerting control over your insulin would then keep mTOR activities within the healthy, muscle-building range. Coupled with exercising and getting your timing right for your meals, you would be able to build muscles more efficiently.

- Taking a break from food may increase your productivity.

    When you do not have to eat, you would be able to allocate the time you have saved from thinking about food to other important activities in your life.

    Rather than worrying about what you are going to eat for lunch or dinner, you may continue working on your projects and tasks. Such concerns are wiped away while you are in a fast.

    Furthermore, once you have gotten control over your hunger pangs, you would notice that concentrating on whatever you are doing becomes easier to sustain. Some researchers suggest that this is linked to the primal part of the human brain.

    Hunger has always been one of the major motivators. Back then, it prompted the early humans to go out and hunt for food. Since hunting requires focus and determination, feelings of hunger become hardwired with our ability to concentrate even when under stressful conditions.

- Fasting keeps the brain healthy and strong.

  Through fasting, the process of autophagy, or the removal of cellular waste, may be activated and sustained. Cleaning up the damaged molecules and cellular components would help you prevent the onset of various neurodegenerative diseases. Furthermore, cleansing the brain can significantly improve its performance and functions.

  Fasting may also boost the production of the BDNF, or the brain-derive neurotrophic factor. This protein keeps the brain cells from dying out due to stressors.

  Studies also show that new connections between your brain cells and tissues may be established quicker through fasting.

- Going through a fast can extend your longevity.

  Ageing impairs your natural cellular stress response. As a result, your cells would begin to degrade and lose their functions over time.

  One of the effective means of warding off the effects of ageing is through the natural rejuvenation processes. Fasting triggers this process since the body recognizes it as an acute stressor.

Moreover, numerous studies have shown that it is actually eating that hastens the process of aging. The increased levels of insulin and mTOR activity causes faster cellular degradation.

Plenty of evidences can be found among cultures that do not encourage overeating. People who are more selective of their foods and beverages tend to live longer and healthier lives.

- Fasting can help you fight off diseases.

Most people naturally feel a loss of appetite whenever they are sick. It may be just a subconscious effort of the body to heal itself, but it is rooted in the fact that fasting can actually help you live a healthier life.

Fasting enables the body to restore the proper pH balance in your blood. As a result, you can prevent the onset of painful ailments of the body, such as arthritis.

It can also improve your control over your insulin levels, thereby improving your resistance towards the following diseases:

- o Diabetes
- o Prostate Cancer
- o Breast Cancer
- o Heart Failure

Fasting has also been found to be effective at reducing both chronic and acute inflammation. When harmful stimuli enter your system, the body would naturally defend itself through an inflammatory reaction. Though they are helpful in keeping you safe, the effects on your body can range from mild pains and redness to serious long-term illnesses, such as:

- Various Forms of Cancer
- Various Forms of Cardiovascular Diseases
- Hypertension
- Diabetes
- Arthritis
  Since inflammation is linked to obesity and overeating, fasting has been identified as a way to control the occurrence of inflammatory reactions across the body.

Fasting will make you feel more energized.

In response to stressful situations, the natural response of the body is to release adrenaline. The higher the stress level, the more fight-or-flight hormones are released into your system. Once your body has entered survival mode, you would feel more alert and ready to act, as expressed in the following signs and symptoms:

o Rapid breathing

o Increased heart rate

o Dilation of the pupils

o Release of fat and glycogen into the bloodstream

Fasting is considered as a mild stressor to the body. Therefore, you would experience the above given signs and symptoms albeit in a lesser degree. Such bodily reactions contribute to the reputation of fasting as an effective means of weight loss.

• When scheduled correctly, fasting can enhance the effects of exercising your body.

Many health experts recommend incorporating exercise routines into a fasting plan. This would enable the body to trigger the detoxification and rejuvenation process. When this occurs, you would experience an increase in the following:

o Lipolysis, or better known as fat burning

o Repair of muscle tissue

o Neurogenesis, or the generation of new brain cells

o Insulin sensitivity

o Cellular stress response

Your body and mind would benefit greatly from a fast. There are also no significant disadvantages for going into fast—as long as you have been given the go signal by your doctor.

Let us take a better look on the subject of insulin and diabetes. Before taking advantage of intermittent fasting, it will be best to understand why it can do more harm than good to have 5-6 meals every day or every few hours (the exact opposite of fasting).

When we consume food, the primary hormone involved in the food we eat is insulin (produced by the pancreas). Both proteins and carbohydrates stimulate insulin. Eating only stimulates a small amount of insulin, but the food is rarely consumed alone.

Insulin has two main functions:

- First, it allows the body to use the energy stemming from the food instantly. Carbohydrates quickly become insulin, which raises the level of blood sugar. Insulin directs glucose to cells in the body for energy use. Proteins are classified into amino acids and sugar surplus amino acids. Protein cannot necessarily raise glucose in our blood but it could stimulate insulin. Fats get a minimal insulin effect.
- The second is that insulin stores excess energy away for future use. In insulin, excess, glucose is transformed into glycogen and stored in the liver. There is an end to how much glycogen can be saved. Once the limit is reached, glucose becomes fat in the liver. The fat is now put away in the liver or fatty deposits in the body (sometimes stored as visceral or belly fat).

- So, if we continuously eat snacks all day long, insulin levels remain high. In other words, we spend most of the day storing food energy.

What happens while we fast?

The process of using and storing the food energy we eat reverses when we are fasting. The levels of insulin drop, and the body starts to burn stored energy. Glycogen is first accessed and uses the glucose that is stored in the liver. The body now starts to break down stored body fat for energy.

The body, therefore, actually resides in two conditions-the fed condition with high insulin and the fasting state with low insulin. Either we store food, or we consume food energy. When dieting and fasting are balanced, there is no change in weight. If we spend most of the day eating and storing energy, we have a good chance of gaining weight over time.

The portion control strategy for constant caloric reduction is the most common dietary recommendation for weight loss and type 2 diabetes. For instance, the American Diabetes Association recommends an energy deficit of 500-750 kcal/day combined with physical activity. Dietitians follow this approach and recommend eating 5-6 small foods all day long.

Does the portion control strategy work over the long term? Rarely. A cohort study of 176,495 obese individuals with a 9 year follow-up UK showed that only 3,528 of them were able to achieve healthy body weight by the end of the trial. This is a 98% failure rate!

Intermittent fasting does not always restrict calories. Restricting calories increases hunger and, worse, causes a reduction in the metabolic rate of the body, a double curse! When we burn fewer calories per day, it becomes even more challenging to lose weight and is easier to regain weight once we have lost it. This type of diet puts the body in a "hunger mode" because metabolism is used to preserve energy.

Intermittent fasting has no such inconvenience.

Health benefits of intermediate fasting include a boost of the metabolism leading to us losing weight and body fat. From a certain point of view, this makes sense. If we don't eat, the body uses stored energy to find another meal to keep us alive. Hormones permit the change of energy sources from food to body fat.

Studies demonstrate this phenomenon. Four days of continuous fasting, for example, increased the base metabolic rate by 12 percent. Norepinephrine, the neurotransmitter that prepares the body for action, was increased by 117%. Fatty acids in the bloodstream rose by more than 370% as the organism changed from oil to fat.

No loss of muscle mass as many fear is caused by intermittent fasting since it does not burn muscles, unlike a consistent, calorie-restricting diet. In 2010, researchers examined a group of subjects who had alternating routine fasting for 70 days (one day and the next). At 52.0 kg, their muscle mass began and ended at 52.9 kg. There is no loss of muscles, but 11.4 percent of fat was lost and high LDL cholesterol and triglyceride levels were increased.

Naturally, the body produces more human growth hormones during fasting to preserve lean muscle and bone. Muscle mass is usually protected until fat falls below 4%. Consequently, most people are not at risk of muscle loss when they do intermittent fasting.

Type 2 diabetes is a condition in which the body has too much sugar to allow cells to respond to insulin and to absorb glucose from their blood (insulin resistance), resulting in high blood sugar. The liver is loaded with fat when trying to clear too much glucose by converting it into fat and saving it with water.

Thus, two things have to happen to reverse this condition-

•   Stop putting more sugar into the body.

•   Second, burn off the rest of the sugar.

A low-carbon, with moderate protein, and a healthy fat diet, also called a ketogenic diet, is the best diet to achieve this. (Remember that carbohydrates increase blood glucose to a maximum level, protein to a certain degree, and fat to a minimum.) This is why a low-carb diet will help reduce incoming glucose burdens. This is already sufficient for some people to reverse insulin resistance and diabetes of type 2. In more severe cases, however, diet alone is not enough.

What about workout? Exercise helps to burn glucose away in the skeletal muscles but not in the fatty liver and all tissues and organs. The task is essential, but to eliminate the excess glucose in the organs, the cells have to be temporarily "starved."

This can be achieved through intermittent fasting. Historically, people have called cleansing or detox fasting. It can be a powerful tool to eliminate all the excesses. It is the quickest way to reduce the level of blood glucose and insulin and to ultimately resist insulin, type 2 diabetes, and fatty liver.

Incidentally, taking insulin for type 2 diabetes does not address the root cause of the body's sugar excess. Insulin will indeed lead to less glucose from the blood, but where does the sugar go? The liver will turn it all into fat, liver fat, and abdominal fat. Insulin patients often gain more weight, which makes their diabetes worse.

Heart health enhancement overtime, high type 2 diabetes and blood glucose can harm the blood vessels and nerves that control the heart. When you have diabetes, the higher the risk is of developing a heart disease. The chances of having a stroke are also reduced by lowering blood sugar and the risk of cardiovascular disease is lowered too.

Furthermore, intermittent fasting, LDL cholesterol, total blood triglycerides, and inflammatory markers associated with many chronic diseases have been demonstrated to improve blood pressure.

Multiple studies showed that fasting has many neurological advantages, including betterment in attention, focus, time of reaction, immediate memory, cognition, and new brain cell generation. Mice studies have also shown that intermittent fasting rapidly reduces brain inflammation and prevents Alzheimer's symptoms.
What to expect with the intermittent fasting of hunger? We usually get hungry for about four hours after we finish a meal. So, if we do not eat for at last 24 hours, will our sense of hunger be six times more severe? Of course not.

Many people worry that fasting will lead to extreme hunger and excessive consumption. Studies have shown that, on the day that follows an abstinence day, the caloric intake rises by 20%. But hunger and appetite decrease surprisingly with repeated fasting.

The starvation comes in waves. If we do nothing, after a while, hunger dissipates. To fight the hunger, it is often enough to drink tea (all sorts) or coffee (with or without caffeine). It is, however, better to drink your coffee black so as to not trigger a large insulin response. Sugar or artificial sweeteners of any kind are not appropriate to use. Bone broth can be consumed during fasting if necessary.

The level of sugar in our blood will not be diminished. Sometimes people worry about their blood sugar levels falling very low resulting in them getting shaky and sweaty during fasting. This does not happen because the body closely monitors blood sugar levels, and multiple mechanisms control it. The body starts breaking down glycogen in the liver during fasting to release glucose. This happens during our sleep every night.

Glycogen stores are perishing when we are fasting for longer than 24-36 hours, and the liver produces new glucose using glycerol as the by-product of the breakup of fat (a process known as gluconeogenesis). The brain can also use ketones for energy, apart from glucose. Ketones are produced when fat is metabolized and can supply up to 75% of the brain's energy demands (the remaining 25% of glucose).

The only exception is for people who take diabetic drugs and insulin. You MUST consult your doctor first, as dosages will probably have to be reduced as you fast. If you do not overmedicate and develop hypoglycemia, this can be dangerous, and you will need to have specific amounts of sugar intake to reverse it. This breaks the fasting and makes it counterproductive.

Many people have high blood glucose after a certain period of fasting, especially in the morning. This dawning is the result of the circadian rhythm, in which the body stores higher levels of several hormones to prepare for the day to come. More specifically:

• Adrenaline-to give the body energy

• Growth hormone-to help repair and create new protein

• Glucagon-to move glucose from liver storage into the blood for use as energy

• Cortisol–stress-hormone–to active protein

• Glucagon - The extent of which is low in non-diabetics, and most people will not even consider it. However, a noticeable rise in blood glucose for most diabetics can occur as the liver dumps sugar into the blood.

This will also happen in long fasts. If there is no food, the level of insulin remains low as the liver releases some of its stored sugar and fat. It's natural and not bad at all. The spike magnitude decreases when the liver is less bloated by sugar and fat.

Fasting may be considered as one of the oldest healing strategies mankind has created.

Chapter 3 – A Brief History of Fasting

There is no point in the known human history wherein the concept of fasting has not existed in some shape or form. The voluntary act of abstaining from eating or drinking has deep roots in different cultures and religions around the world. Each type may vary at some point or another, but the core principles of fasting remain the same.

Fasting is as old as humanity, much older than any other type of diet. Ancient civilizations, like the Greeks, have recognized the intrinsic benefit of periodic fasting. These were often referred to as cycles of treatment, purification, and detox. Almost every culture and religion on earth perform certain fasting rituals.

Before the introduction of agriculture, people never ate three meals a day plus snacks. We only ate when we found food that could be separated by hours or days. Thus, from an evolutionary point of view, eating three meals a day is not a survival requirement. Perhaps, as a species, we would not have survived.

We have all forgotten this ancient practice before the 21st century. Fasting is bad for business, after all! Food producers allow us to eat snacks and multiple meals a day. Nutrition authorities warn against the severe effects of skipping a single meal. These messages have been drilled in our heads over time.

Even the motivations behind each variation tend to be of similar natures. For some, fasting is a way to heal the body and the mind. Most religions, on the other hand, believe it is a way of strengthening the spirit and one's connection to a divine being.

To better illustrate the universality of fasting across time and location, here are the important historical highlights that would give you a better picture of the practice of fasting across different cultures and religions.

- One of the earliest records of fasting show that a number of prominent ancient Greek figures were believers. For example, Pythagoras, a legendary Greek philosopher and mathematician, followed a 40-day starvation cycle in order to enhance his creativity and mental clarity.

The father of modern medicine, Hippocrates, was among the first to recognize the applications of fasting to the medical field. His observations of the human body had led him to a conclusion that a sick body would benefit from the absence of food.

Ancient Greek healers had also observed that the frequency of epileptic seizures was lower among patients who were engaging in a fast at the time compared to those who were not.

- Some ancient cultures, such as the Natives from North America, believed that fasting before a war would ensure their success in battle. They had also engaged in fasting to prevent the occurrence of wide-scale catastrophes like famine and drought.

- Both the Old Testament and the New Testament of the Bible mention several instances of fasting. Even Jesus Christ himself had fasted for 40 days and 40 nights in a desert. Other Biblical figures who have also fasted include Moses, Elijah, and Paul, one of Jesus' apostles.

Given its presence in the Bible, the Christian church encourages its followers to participate in a 40-day fast before Easter as a form of repentance. Though the exact date on which this practice had first been adapted is unknown, the fasting guidelines imposed among Christians have become more lenient throughout the years.

- Muslims practice fasting since it is one of the Five Pillars of Islam—the others being (1) pilgrimage, (2) prayer, (3) declaration of faith, and (4) charity. They believe that through fasting, they would become closer to Allah because it begins with a spiritual intention. Furthermore, fasting fosters solidarity among Muslims who are also fasting, and amplifies feelings of compassion and empathy towards those who are suffering.

These beliefs culminate during Ramadan, a Muslim holiday that is characterized by a month-long period of fasting. During this time, all Muslims are prohibited from consuming food while there is daylight.

- Buddhist monks and nuns abide by the rules of Vinyana, wherein it is stated that followers should not eat anything after they had taken their meals at noon. However, the followers themselves do not consider this as a form of fasting. Instead, they think of it as a part of their normal routine.

- The fasting days among Hindus differ depending on which deity they are following. For example, Vishnu requires fasting on a Thursday, while followers of Shiva fast on a Monday. Hindus also engage in monthly fasting periods that occur after certain lunar phases.

  There are also individuals who perform complete or partial fasting as part of a religious practice called Vratas. Aside from abstaining from food and/or water, those who are practicing it are required to observe personal hygiene, celibacy, and honesty, among others.

- The traditional form of Judaism includes a requirement of 6 fasting days within a given year among its followers. The fasting day lasts from sunset of a particular day up to the sunset of the succeeding day.

- Jains believe that fasting regulates the demands of their bodies, eliminates their accumulated bad karma, and rejuvenates their spirits. As such, they make it a point to incorporate fasting into their day to day lives. Aside from abstaining from food and water, Jains are also required to worship their gods, serve Jain monks and nuns, and engage in acts of charity while fasting.

- A secular fasting holiday in Geneva, Switzerland called the "Jeune Genevois" originated in the Middle Ages. During that period, the people dedicated certain days of the year for fasting as a form of penitence whenever they experienced epidemics, wars, and other big-scale calamities.

As shown through these examples of fasting traditions, fasting has been in existence for hundreds of years, and will continue to be practiced across the world in the foreseeable future.

Fasting has also undergone evolution throughout the years. Though most practitioners perform it as a part of their religious beliefs, a growing number of health enthusiasts have recognized the benefits of fasting on their health.

If you are not fasting due to your religion, then you may still practice fasting according to your current lifestyle, personal preferences, and fitness goals. To guide you through this, the next section of this book covers the various modern ways of fasting that you may consider doing.

Chapter 4 – Discovering the Various Ways to Fast

There is no universal way to fast that could work for everybody. Instead, you get to choose from various methods depending on how much commitment you can give, your personal fitness goals, and your lifestyle preferences. Some involve 24-hour fasting periods. Shorter ones typically last from 12 to 16 hours.

The level of dietary strictness also differs from method to another. Some methods do not allow the follower to consume anything except for water, while controlled fasts aim to only reduce your daily caloric intake.

To guide you in selecting the right fasting method for you, here is a rundown of the effective options that most people choose:

- Intermittent Fasting

  This is one of the simplest fasting methods to apply into your lifestyle. All you need to do is take a break from eating for 24 hours once or twice per week.

  By doing so, you would be able to significantly decrease your calorie intake for the given week, without having to keep track of the calorie count of every single item that you are going to consume. You are not obliged to make any big changes to your lifestyle and diet during your non-fasting days.

To help you assess the potential of intermittent fasting as the ideal fasting protocol for you, here are its pros over the other methods discussed in this book.

- o You are free to adjust your fasting schedule according to your preferences.

   The day and timing of your fasting does not matter as long as you do it on a weekly basis. Some people prefer doing intermittent fasting during the weekends, while some have an easier time doing it on weekdays.

   Pick the best day and time for you so that you would be more successful in sticking with intermittent fasting. Just avoid drawing it beyond the suggested 24-hour fasting period to prevent the occurrence of any health complications.

- o You may use your fasting day to engage in fulfilling and more productive activities.

   Taking a break from eating, even for just a day, would give you more opportunities to pursue other worthwhile activities. For one day per week, you are free from having to prepare and cook your meals, or think about where you are going to eat.

o You can save more money from your weekly budget allocation for food.

Because you are not going to eat during certain times and days of the week, you would be able to reduce your weekly grocery bill.

It is also important for you to recognize the downsides of intermittent fasting before making a decision. For your guidance, here are the known cons of this fasting method.

o The 24-hour duration may be too difficult to observe, especially among beginners.

If you have not experienced fasting before, you are likely going to feel disoriented by the common side-effects of intermittent fasting, such as having low energy for a significant portion of your fasting day. Some people also experience a hard time in staving off their hunger.

○ It may take you a while before you can get accustomed to the negative effects of intermittent fasting on your body.

You can eventually overcome these challenges, provided that you would practice proper intermittent fasting on a regular basis.

Some experts suggest taking baby steps before taking on the full 24-hour duration of this method. At the very least, you should aim to fast for 22 hours in order to reap the benefits of intermittent fasting.

Though you cannot eat anything during your fasting period, you are allowed to drink zero-calorie drinks throughout the day. The most important of these drinks is plain water, which can keep hunger at bay while helping you stay hydrated.

Though certain coffees and teas are also allowed, you should try to limit them as much as possible. At most, you should be drinking only two cups of a caffeinated beverage during your fasting day.

You would also have to break your fast the right way. Some beginners make the mistake of eating unhealthy foods once they have completed a 24-hour fasting period. To prevent you from committing the same mistake, here is a list of foods that you may eat after fasting:

- o Raw vegetable slices, such as fresh carrots, cucumber, broccoli, and celery

- o Hard-boiled eggs

- o Unsalted nuts, such as cashews and walnuts

Try to have these post-fast snacks ready before even going into a fast. Heading to the grocery store during or right after you're finishing your fast would only cause you to buy more foods than you actually need. You might also be tempted to buy certain food products that look appealing but are not exactly healthy choices for you.

Health experts also recommend taking dietary supplements while you are engaged in intermittent fasting. Your options include multivitamins, fish oil, and other common supplements that you normally take while you are not on a fast.

In terms of beverages, you should stick to pure water, unsweetened tea, black coffee, and other zero-calorie beverages. There are several diet beverages out there that claim to be good for your health. Avoid them at all cost because they might contain harmful chemicals that could negatively affect your health.

In fact, even non-caloric artificial sweeteners, such as aspartame and stevia, are highly discouraged among people who are engaged in fasting. You should be giving your body a break from these chemicals, especially since you are putting more strain on your body while you are in a fast.

- Extended Fasting

  Fasting that goes beyond the 24-hour period is considered by health experts as extended fasting. There are several sub-types of this fasting protocol.

  At its most extreme, a person would have to abstain from both food and water during the entirety of the long-term fasting period. Referred to as the dry fast, this method is not advisable for most people, especially since going for more than one day without a drink can cause serious harm to the body.

  Another common sub-form of extended fasting is water fasting. This simply means that you can drink water and other zero-calorie beverages during the extended fasting period. Some experts allow the consumption of juice and broths as well, but others do not because both fluids contain calories and nutrients that can slow down your progress.

Extended fasting has a number of advantages and benefits that might make it the top choice for you. To help you determine if this is the right method for you, here are its known pros.

o You may use this to completely break free from unhealthy eating habits.

    Many people who undergo extended fasting tend to have a spiritual or religious reason for doing so. Even if you are not doing it for similar reasons, you may follow their example by incorporating meditation during your extended fasting periods. This would enable you to contemplate fully what you are embarking on, and what you want to achieve from your fast.

    In the process, you would have the opportunity to reset your relationship with food. If you tend to eat according to your emotions, then the extended fasting may help you get rid of that bad habit. Take note, however, that it is not, by any

means, a miracle cure for any form
of eating disorder.

o   You are going to burn more body fat.

Extended fasting allows your body to
remain in ketosis for a longer period
of time. As a result, your body would
have to unlock your stored body fats,
and convert them into useable forms
of energy.

Remaining in ketosis is essential in
rapid weight loss because it can also
suppress your hunger—that is, as
long as you can successfully get
through the fasting stage.

Not a lot of beginners choose extended
fasting as their first fasting protocol,
primarily because of the following
reasons.

o   Committing to an extended fast can
be intimidating and overwhelming,
especially for beginners.

Going for a fast for more than a day
takes a lot of mental fortitude and
determination—something   that
beginners   might   not   naturally
possess. Abstaining from food and
water for long periods of time can be
daunting, particularly when your
former lifestyle is far from healthy.

If you are set on going through an extended fast, you must allow yourself to get acquainted first with the ins and outs of fasting. Taking small but gradual steps will help you prepare your body and mind for the time when you have to put them under great strain during an extended fast.

o You are putting yourself at serious risk if you do not implement and control it well.

The ultimate risk of extended fasting is death by starvation, dehydration, or both. You should be well attuned with the signals of your body to keep yourself from harm during an extended fasting. Learning when to quit is just as important as being brave enough to push through the challenges of extended fasting.

Since you are not going to eat anything during an extended fast, what you should be mindful about instead are the foods that you can eat when you have to break your fast. This is critical because gorging yourself with the wrong kinds of food after an extended fast would only lead you to regaining most of the weight you have lost during the fasting period.

Here is a set of guidelines that you should observe when breaking your extended fast:

o Your first meals should either be bone broths or fruit juices that have been diluted with water. These are both high in electrolytes, which your body needs the most at this point. It is best if you can make it yourself. However, if that is not possible, then make sure that what you have bought from the store is free from sugar and artificial additives.

o Introduce solid foods into your diet after a couple of days. However, the actual adjustment period depends on how long you have engaged in extended fasting. In general, the longer your fast is, the more time you need to prepare your body for solid foods.

o Soups are excellent dishes that you can eat to make the transition to solid foods easier. Opt for vegetable soups first before going for those with meats in them.

o Avoid eating fruits during your transition period. Though they are soft enough to cause less strain on your digestive system, the amount of fructose is not advisable for your body that has just exited a fasted state.

o Avoid the urge to overeat in order to satisfy your hunger. You must also take your time so that your digestive system would be able to better digest your food.

- The 5:2 Diet

More commonly known as the Fast Diet, this method is considered by many experts as the best way to introduce your body to the principle of controlled fasting. Most followers of this diet also use this as a way to gradually increase their tolerance for the negative side-effects of fasting on them.

For this diet, you would have to limit your calorie intake by consuming only two meals for two days out of a given week. This means that your body would be in a fasted state for about 12 to 16 hours, depending on how you are going to structure your fasting days.

To better understand this method, here are the pros of going into the 5:2 Diet:

o You will never have to fast for a whole day.

Many beginners may feel intimated by the requirements of other fasting methods, especially those that require full-day fasting periods.

With the 5:2 diet, you would never have to go on a fast for more than 12 hours per day. As long as you perform it twice a week, you would be able to feel its positive effects on your body.

o You are free to choose your preferred fasting day within a given week.

Given the mechanics of this diet, you may be able to make it your own. Assess yourself to discover which days of the week, and times of the day would be the most appropriate for your needs and preferences.

Many people try to avoid fasting on two consecutive days. Leaving at least one day in between each fasting period would allow you to recover from the physical, mental, and emotional strain that may be brought about by fasting.

If you have any obligations or engagements that would conflict with your pre-set fasting schedule, you may alter it accordingly. Again, your primary objective is to fast two times per week. The exact schedule would not affect the outcome that you may expect from this method.

o You can enjoy eating your favorite food without feeling guilty about it.

Since you are only required to fast for two days in a week, you may eat normally for the remaining five days.

Do not, however, give in to the temptation to overcompensate for the meals that you have missed during your fasting period. Otherwise, you would be defeating the purpose of going through the 5:2 diet.

o There are no complicated rules to follow.

The rules for this diet are simple enough, even for complete novices. All you have to do is limit your calorie intake during your two-day fasting period.

Like other methods, there are some disadvantages to choosing the 5:2 Diet. For example:

o You will never experience the benefits of a full-day fast.

Since you are still going to consume food during your fasting day, your blood sugar level would still rise up to a certain level. When this occurs, the fat-burning activities within your body would come to a halt.

o You may feel hungrier than usual while you are fasting.

Some people also report feelings of intense starvation in the middle of their fasting period because they are coming down from the rise of blood sugar that they have experienced right after the meal.

Since the 5:2 Diet allows you to eat meals even during your fasting days, you should be extra mindful of your food choices. As a general rule, you should stick to foods that are highly nutritious but have low GI scores. Such foods would make you feel fuller for longer periods of time while keeping your blood sugar at manageable levels.

You should also opt for high-protein foods since they take longer to digest. In terms of carbohydrates, you should limit yourself only to complex variants rather than simple ones, such as white bread, cookies, and other pastries.

What you eat on non-fasting days also matters in the 5:2 Diet. First, do not think of them as eat-anything-you-want days. Do not also try to make up for the calorie deficit during your fasting day. Going for extra helpings during lunch or dinner would set you back a couple of steps away from your goal.

- Alternate-Day Fasting

  As its name suggests, the general principle behind this method is going on a fast every other day. In its most basic form, you would be allowed to drink only zero-calorie drinks during your fasting days.

  Some forms, however, permit the consumption of meals that do not exceed the 500-calorie limit. Whichever the case may be, as long as you are fasting every other day, then you are engaging in the alternate-day fasting method.

  Here are the pros of choosing this strategy:

  o You only have to fast half of the time.

    Compared to other fasting methods that must be done on a daily basis in order to have an impact on your health, the mechanics of the alternate-fasting enables you to live and eat as you normally do on your off-days.

Remember to keep things on the healthy side, however, because reverting back to processed food and sugary beverages during your break from fasting would be detrimental to the overall success of this method.

○ It is more effective at preserving your muscle mass compared to the other fasting methods.

Normally, the rate of fat-burning within your body is directly correlated to the loss of muscle mass. As such, those who are hoping to obtain leaner muscles through a fast may find it hard to maintain the muscle tissues that they have developed through exercising.

On the other hand, studies show that those who the alternate-day fasting manage to maintain their muscle mass even though they have lost more body fat than those who belong to other test groups. Therefore, if you are aiming to build your muscles while you are losing your excess weight, then the most appropriate method for you may be the alternate-day fasting.

o It can trigger the process of autophagy.

Autophagy plays a critical role in removing the damaged components from your cells and organ systems. Through this process, you would be able to significantly lessen your chances of developing serious chronic illnesses, such as cancer, cardiovascular diseases, and various types of bodily infections.

The problem is that it does not automatically occur, unless it is triggered. One way to do so is by adapting the alternate-day fasting. Researchers have found out that through this method, you would be able to reduce the damage in your body caused by oxidation. As a result, this could also increase your longevity in the process of cleansing your body from within.

To even things out, here are the cons of the alternate-day fasting that you have to consider:

o Due to the fasting schedule of this method, it may take a while before you can get used to being in a fasted state.

Some people consider the lack of continuity per day as the reason for their slow adjustment towards the changes in their life caused by fasting. This pertains more on the negative side-effects such as more frequent hunger pangs, lightheadedness, and low energy levels.

Since you only have to undergo fasting every other day, your body and mind may not become acclimatized to fasting within the expected one to two-week adjustment period.

○ The weight loss effects of alternate-day fasting may not be as quick as the other fasting methods.

Again, since you are not restricting your calorie intake during your off-days, you might notice that you are not shedding off your excess weight, especially during the first few times you have implemented this method.

As verified by multiple studies, the amount of body fat that you may lose through fasting tends to be compounded by the water weight that you also lose during a fast. This water weight, unlike body fat, can be easily regained whenever you consume foods without exercising at all.

To keep you on track with your weight loss goals while following the alternate-day fasting, you should increase your exercise during your off-days. This would enable you to exert control over the possibility of regaining your water weight.

You should also be mindful of the meal restrictions for alternate day fasting.

o If you are following a sub-form of this method where you are allowed to eat, you should eat meals and snacks that would not total up to more than 500 calories per day.

Therefore, you should go for highly nutritious yet filling foods, such as organic vegetables, lean meats, and fish.

o In order to feel full despite the lower calories, you should include more soup into your meal plan. Salads with generous helpings of lean meat may also be a good option for you, especially during your off days.

○ For drinks, you should stick to low-calorie or zero-calorie beverages, such as water, herbal tea, and black coffee.

- Micro-Fasting

Unlike methods that advocate for longer fasting period, micro-fasting may be done on a daily basis. Most of its followers simply think of this as the no-breakfast diet, because you have to be in a fasted state for 16 hours every day, thus compressing your feeding periods to 8 hours per day only.

Almost half of the 16-hour fasting period is done while you are asleep, and you continue it from the moment you wake up until lunch time, where you can have your first meal of the day.

The main principle behind this method is controversial, especially given the importance placed by some health experts on breakfast. However, multiple studies have demonstrated that micro-fasting does not cause any of the ill effects expected from regularly skipping breakfasts.

There are various pros for doing a micro-fast, as explained below:

o The shorter fasting duration of this method may be easier for you.

This method is highly suggested for those who cannot or do not want to engage in a 24-hour fast. At most, you would have to abstain from food for only 16 hours per day.

o More frequent fasting periods tend to be more effective for many people.

Studies show that the more you micro-fast, the more benefits you may get from doing it. Extended fasting periods are not always better than shorter, but more frequent bouts of fasting.

After all, you have to maintain the delicate balance between feeding and fasting in order to attain and sustain optimum health.

o You can set the timing of your workouts after engaging in micro-fasting.

Exercising right after a fasting period significantly enhances the positive effects of physical activities on your health.

When you get the timing right, you would lose more weight and feel more energized after exercising.

○ It is more flexible compared to other fasting methods.

Even though many experts suggest the daily practice of micro-fasting, you are not required to do it every day.

Therefore, you are free to choose which days you are going to engage in a fast, and which days would be dedicated to your other important activities.

○ You may still join others and socialize with them during meal times.

Some people hesitate in committing to intermittent fasting because it is hard and awkward to socialize during lunch time or dinner time when they are not eating like their companions do.

Micro-fasting only requires you to skip breakfast and refrain from having snacks after dinner. You are then free to eat the rest of your meals with your family, friends, or co-workers.

To set the right expectations for micro-fasting, you should also be aware of the cons of choosing this fasting method.

o The positive effects of fasting may be reduced.

According to multiple research studies on fasting, most of the benefits that you may expect from intermittent fasting can be obtained within the initial 12 to 16 hours of a fasting period. You would then get the rest of the benefits, such as increased fat-burning rate, and more growth hormones during the last 8 hours of a fast.

Since micro-fasting only lasts for 16 hours per day, you may not be able to reap the full benefits of intermittent fasting.

o The increased frequency of fasting periods may pose a challenge to you.

Some people find it harder to micro-fast every day than to fast for 24 hours once or twice per week.

Ultimately, this depends on your lifestyle, current responsibilities, and personal preferences.

o You cannot eat your breakfast.

Perhaps one of the most controversial aspects of micro-fasting is its rule against eating breakfast.

Many health experts consider breakfast as the most important meal of the day. However, some studies show that you do not necessarily need breakfast to boost your energy and productivity for the rest of the day.

Compared to other forms of fasting method, the timing of your meals during a micro-fast is a critical factor that you have to get right. Otherwise, it would be hard for you to stave off hunger for the rest of the day.

The optimal timing varies from one person to another, but for your reference, here is a list of the common eight-hour window times that you may consider following:

o   10:00 AM to 6:00 PM
o   11:00 AM to 7:00 PM
o   12:00 Noon to 8:00 PM
o   1:00 PM to 9:00 PM
o   2:00 PM to 10:00 PM

Check which of these time periods would work best with the rest of your schedule for the day. By doing so, micro-fasting would not have to be a burden onto you and the people around you.

Since you have to skip breakfast, you must make your first meal of the day the biggest one that you will eat for that given day. Aside from giving you an energy boost, it would also increase the amount of food that your digestive system can process and absorb at a time.

However, do not eat until you are completely stuffed. Aim for a feeling of satisfaction instead.

Since you are limiting the amount of calories that you can eat, you should also take extra care about the kinds of food that you are eating. As much as possible, your diet should consist mostly of organic fruits and vegetables. These foods have the highest level of calorie-to-nutrient ratio.

For proteins, it is best to stick with fishes, lean meats, and poultry. In terms of carbohydrates, your body would benefit more from complex carbohydrates such as sweet potatoes and whole grains.

As mentioned earlier, exercising is a critical part of micro-fasting. Therefore, you should try to exercise first before eating meal. This will help your body to redirect the nutrition from the meal you have eaten into the development of your muscles rather. Otherwise, most of your nutrients would be stored as body fats.

It is best to limit your exercises to only 5-minute sessions. Each session must be intense, however, in order to unlock the benefits of exercising before eating your meal. Examples of brief but intense exercises that you do include sprinting and lifting heavy weights.

- The Warrior Diet

This method bears striking similarities with micro-fasting, especially when it comes to limiting your feeding periods. Specifically, the Warrior Diet only allows its followers to eat during a four-hour window time in the evening.

The restrictions during the 20-hour fasting period are less strict, however, than micro-fasting. In this regard, the Warrior Diet appears to be more like a type of controlled fast. A person is allowed to eat raw or live foods during the earlier parts of the fasting period within a given day. This is then followed by an overeating phase during the latter part of the same day.

It may be an unconventional form of fasting for some, but many of its followers find it to be effective and even satisfying to a certain point.

To help you decide whether or not this is the right fasting method for you, here are the pros of the Warrior Diet compared to other forms of fasting strategies.

o You may eat light foods throughout the day.

Unlike other methods that limit you to fluids only during the fasting periods, the Warrior Diet allows the consumption of live or raw foods whenever you feel intense hunger pangs that cannot be relieved by a simple drink.

As such, it may be more suitable for those who cannot fully commit to a no-food fasting diet.

o It is beneficial to the improvement of your brain health.

The Warrior Diet would help you regulate the inflammatory pathways that are linked to several types of neurodegenerative diseases, such as Alzheimer's disease. Studies also show that it can reduce the likelihood of brain tumors that may be detrimental to your capacity to learn and memorize things.

Like other forms of fasting, there are also some cons to choosing the Warrior Diet. For example:

o Changing your lifestyle to suit the standards of this diet can be quite challenging.

This applies for both beginners and more experienced individuals. For instance, unlike in micro-fasting, the period for undereating lasts longer than the standard 16-hour fasting period.

You do get to eat one full and hearty meal per day, but some people find it hard to stick to this rule.

Furthermore, studies show that being allowed to eat lightly makes it harder to get through a fasting period compared to completely abstaining from food.

o It is not recommended for certain groups of people.

Due to the limited window of time for eating, the Warrior Diet may not be suitable for children, pregnant or nursing mothers, high-level athletes, people with eating disorders, and people who are underweight.

Recent studies also show that the Warrior Diet may alter the hormonal balance among women. Granted that other forms of fasting method may also cause this, the effect of the Warrior Diet among women tend to be more pronounced than the rest. For example, some women may begin suffering from irregular menstrual cycles, and anxiety as a side-effect of going through the Warrior Diet.

The Warrior Diet involves two phases: undereating and overeating. It is important for you to learn which foods you can consume for each phase.

The undereating period would take up most of your day. The general rule during this phase is to impose strict limits upon what and how much you can eat.

Health experts recommend eating only fresh produce and a bit of light protein. You can turn the raw fruits and vegetables into juices as well, if that would be more appealing to you.

Here is a list of acceptable foods that you can eat during the undereating phase:

o Carrot sticks
o A handful of blueberries, strawberries, or raspberries
o Unsweetened coconut water
o Plain water
o Black coffee
o Unsweetened tea
o Small cups of yoghurt
o A couple of eggs
o Low-salt, homemade broths

Once the undereating phase has reached its end, you will be entering the overeating period. As its name suggests, you would have to eat more than you normally do. The main restriction is that you can only do so for one meal during your four-hour feeding time in the evening.

To overeat, you must consume foods until you feel full. You do not have to think about the exact number of calories that you are consuming since this method wants you to tap into your primal eating instincts.

However, you should still limit yourself to only healthy foods since processed food products and junk foods would be detrimental to your overall well-being.

Here is a list of the kinds of food that you should eat during the overeating phase:

- o Salads made of green leafy vegetables and lean proteins

- o Dense carbohydrates, such as root crops and whole grains

- o Healthy fats, like ghee, natural butter, and unsalted nuts

Keep in mind that overeating is only considered as okay because you are consuming a lot of healthy foods. Some people assume that calories are bad for you, whether or not they come from good sources. However, various studies conducted on the effectivity of the Warrior Diet proves that this belief is not a solid fact.

Figuring out the best way to fast is mostly a matter of your personal preference. Each of the above given fasting methods work, though every method has some benefits that are unique to them.

Remember, there is no single method that is objectively better than the other. What would set apart your choice from the rest is your capacity to remain committed to your selected method. Assess yourself versus the pros and cons of each method to get a better idea of which of these methods would fit best with your lifestyle and goals.

Chapter 5 – What to Expect When Starting to Fast

Setting your expectations before committing to a fast is an excellent way of preparing both your body and mind for the lifestyle and dietary changes that are about to happen.

Before delving into the details of these expectations, you should be clear first about your personal objectives for the fast. Here are some common scenarios that have led people into fasting:

- They want to lose weight, and gain a leaner body.

- They have tried other popular diets before, and they felt dissatisfied with the process, or frustrated over the results.

- They want to significantly improve the current condition of their body.

- They want to live a longer, healthier, and more productive life.

Fasting is a proven method of losing weight in a healthy manner, while increasing your energy levels. For many, it is a life-changing practice that has enabled them to achieve their other personal goals in life.

Committing to a fast requires determination and confidence that you can go through this without giving in to your old ways. You need to plan and prepare for this because you might have to make drastic changes in your life.

For your guidance, here are the various things that you should expect when starting a fast:

- Grocery Shopping

  Fasting would significantly change the way you shop for food. Aside from the frequency of your shopping days, some items from your current shopping list must be removed and replaced with healthier alternatives.

  In general, you should stick to leaner types of proteins, such as certain types of fishes and egg whites. For fruits and vegetables, it is advisable to spend a bit more and buy organic produce.

- Meal Restrictions

  The exact meal schedule that you have to observe depends on the fasting method that you are following. However, all fasting methods would limit your calorie intake either by reducing the allowable number of calories, or by urging you to skip certain meals—if not all of them.

For example, a 5:2 diet imposes a 500-calorie limit among women, and 600-calorie limit among men. Both are significantly less than the recommended amount for average individuals.

Imbibing alcohol drinks during a fast is strongly discouraged as well. Even when you are on your "off days" from your fast, experts recommend only a moderate amount.

During a fast, you would also have to drink more water. If you prefer flavored beverages, then you should stick to herbal teas and black coffee with no sugar. Some health experts also allow drinking club soda during a fast.

Refer to chapter 4 of this book for more information about the meal restrictions of different fasting methods.

- Physiological side-effects

  Many of these side-effects can be considered as the disadvantages of fasting. However, with the right mindset, you would be able to power through them despite the challenges they might pose to your day-to-day life.

  o   Hunger Pangs

Hunger is a natural reaction of the body when you begin abstaining from food. It is an unavoidable aspect of fasting, but it is not entirely a negative one. Studies show that hunger can actually increase your focus and improve your mental clarity.

o Lightheadedness

It may take you some time to get used to being in a fasted state. During your adjustment period, you are likely going to experience lightheadedness and other uncomfortable bodily sensations. Those are perfectly normal, and they will go away once your body has fully adapted to the changes in your lifestyle.

o Low Energy

Experiencing a drop in your energy levels is another short-term symptom that you should expect and prepare for during the initial stages of your fast.

Your body is used to getting a certain amount of calories per day. When you begin skipping your meals, your body would have to adjust and trigger other internal processes that could provide you the energy you need to perform normally.

According to experts, this period of low energy can last from one to two weeks. After that, you would be able to feel more energized even when you continue being in a fasted state.

Learning how to prepare yourself for this positive change in your life is important. It's best to switch to a low-carbohydrate, fatty diet for three weeks if anyone wants to start intermittent fasting. It allows the body to use fat rather than sugar as an energy source. This involves the removal of all sugars, cereals (bread, cookies, pasta, rice), vegetables, and refined oils. This will minimize the most fasting side effects.

Start with a shorter pace of 16 hours, for instance, from dinner (8 pm) to lunch the next day (12 pm). You will usually eat between 12 and 20 pm and consume two or three meals. You can extend it quickly to 18, 20 hours once you feel comfortable with it.

For shorter fasts, you can do so continuously every day. You can do it 1-3 times a week for more prolonged fasts, such as 24-36 hours, alternating between fasting and regular eating days.

To better illustrate what you would go through during a fast, here is an overview of a typical intermittent and extended fasting period.

- Your body will enter its fasting state at around 8 hours after your last meal. This is the average duration for a full digestion and complete absorption of nutrients from the food and beverages you have consumed prior to your fasting period.

  It could vary, however, depending on the kind of meal you had—for instance, foods high in fiber need a longer digestive period compared to leafy vegetables.

- During the initial fasting period, your body would still get most of its energy from your glucose stores, or also known as glycogen.

- The glycogen stored in your liver would be depleted after an overnight fast.

- Once completely your body has completely used up all the glucose stores in your body, it would begin sourcing energy from the fat stores within your body.

  Take note, however, that the body is already converting fat into energy even before you have consumed all the glycogen in your body. Fasting only increases the rate of fat-burning, thus making it an effective means of losing excess weight.

There's no right fasting scheme. The essential thing is to choose one that works best for you. Some people get results with shorter fasts; others may require longer fasts. Some people make classic water-just fast; others make tea and coffee quickly, others a bone broth. Regardless of what you do, keeping hydrated, and monitoring yourself is very important. You should stop immediately if you feel ill at any point. You might be hungry, but don't feel sick.

Knowing what to expect is critical in the long-term success of your fast. Realign your goals based on what you have learned from this chapter so that you can create a realistic and achievable fasting plan.

Chapter 6 – The Weight Loss Effects of Fasting: Drawbacks and Benefits

To desire the rapid benefits of fasting, we first need to understand the concept of rapid weight loss.

So, what's fasting? It merely is the method of intentionally abstaining (with the exception of water) from food and drink for some time.

Fasts have been used for many centuries and have become very common in the last few years, particularly fasting for weight loss. The explanation for this was based on a case study without high expectations, with people who had to participate in it for a year. They expected nothing from this study, but the findings were so good, a more in-depth analysis was needed.

With rapid benefits, people have naturally lost weight and improved their health problems. You will look younger and have a happier and longer life! This is why you will find this approach so appealing. Honestly, this diet is not that difficult. Basically, what you're doing is eating for 24 hours and then fasting for the next 24 hours. Water is allowed, of course. It differs significantly from our usual eating habits. Although it may seem to be an extreme weight loss process, fasting to lose weight is supported by science as the most successful and natural way out!

Here are the three most effective intermittent fasting methods for weight loss:

Detoxification-One of the most significant speed benefits of all. You quickly experience a self-cleaning process, free from the constant processing of meat. This allows you to wipe out your accumulated body toxins during heavy lunches or fast foods. And then, you feel great!

Developing tolerance-Most people tend to ignore this significant rapid gain. Unfortunately, most of us, lack this vital quality not only during our dieting but also in daily life. Patience comes from exercising self-control. Think of it as a muscle: the more you exercise it, the stronger it becomes. And, together with other fasting benefits, you will also become mentally stronger!

Significant loss of weight-Naturally! Today, this is the biggest fasting benefit, and the main reason why most people get into it is to lose weight quickly. In reality, as it happened in the long past, our bodies are designed to live long without food. The muscles and liver store energy as glycogen while we eat. During fasting period the body starts to burn off the fat and uses glycogen.

These rapid advantages are only the basic ones. The truth of the matter is that besides these general benefits, each person enjoys different gains from the fasting procedure based on their body type and personality. Do not forget that every one of us needs to be in the shape he or she desires to be!

Keep in mind that intermittent fasting is a new way of eating which only recently gained the attention it deserves. All of us have been advised that one must exercise regularly and with a lot of fervor to lose weight. While this is true, the fact that daily exercise is essential to maintain a healthy outlook and burn fat, is it enough? It is impossible to lose weight without dietary changes and maintaining those changes consistently. Most people are giving up on their diets and exercise because conventional wisdom says that you must take away the foods you enjoy to lose weight.

But what if you don't?

Intermittent weight loss fasting is not necessarily a new phenomenon. Fasting is a daily part of life in many countries, both for educational and religious purposes. In such situations, fasting is not performed for weight loss but to cleanse the skin. In most cases, this fasting method lasts from several days to a month.

What if they eat every day instead of fasting for days? Alternate methods for rapid weight loss do just that. Instead of fasting for weeks, the practitioner fasts for about 16-20 hours every day.

A typical food day for most people is something like the following:

8:00 am. Breakfast 11:00 am — dinner at 6:00 pm.

This schedule means eating is spread through a 12-hour eating window, allowing you to eat relatively the same amounts of food in a compressed timeframe for a considerable amount of time during intermittent fasts. The irregular schedule for fasting weight loss would seem to be the following:

8:00 am Breakfast - 1:00 pm Lunch - 6:00 pm Dinner

What we have done above is to limit the meal window to eight hours. Nothing but water should be consumed outside the 8-hour window. This has several significant advantages. First of all, you will eat less since most people do not digest their food fast enough to eat the same amount of food they would eat under different circumstances.

Eating less food and using the same amount of daily exercise will be equal to losing weight.

The body has more chances of flushing excess salt and waste because more water is absorbed.

Does fasting intermittently work?

Definitely. Absolutely. You can use it to drop fat consistently while maintaining your muscle mass and gain strength. There is a timeframe of about two weeks to adjust to this schedule. During this time your body and mind are getting used to the food changes. After two weeks, hunger cravings will begin to fade.

The inexperienced authors can usually be identified by their opening statements, which generally consist of a positive remark and an important question. The most frequent lead-in appears to have been: "Fasting has been practiced worldwide for centuries... but can it help prevent a disease? Doing it helps you lose weight and makes you healthier?" The truth is, it is not a procedure to practice; it is a decision to take.

Is it a fast and easy thing? No, and this is true for several reasons. Most Americans are accustomed to eating. Most prefer eating to abstain for a while and cleanse their organism. Many are too fond of food and cherish it as much as their life. If someone misses a meal, what would you expect them to say? "I am extremely hungry!" Americans need to have food inside their belly for 24 hours a day. Most of them have never heard about the word' fast'. Those who have heard about it think it is merely an exercise most commonly found in religion. Those who are pro fasting recommend it only for a few days, or they plan fasting with juice rather than with water;

1.   Is fasting safe for weight loss?
2.   Is it possible to significantly improve severe medical conditions by fasting?
3.   Is it safe to fast?
4.   Will quickness provide longevity?

Weight loss through fasting is a useful weight-loss tool? To answer the first question we must first understand what the rapidity is, what's involved, how our body responds to it, and what the specific length which we can expect is results.

- Does the subject have food disorders, addictions to food, including medicines or alcohol?
- How is the health of the matter? (They should be under medical supervision, should they be questionable.)
- What is their age? (under 18, parental and or medical supervision should be necessary.)
- How long is the speed?
- What are your expectations? (It is essential to set a lower reasonable goal.) (What do you hope to achieve physically and mentally?)
- Do you work fast? (Home or work?)
- Do they have family and friends support?

These are concerns and questions that a health professional should answer for you. Sadly, the lack of educated, skilled people in the field of healthcare and preventive medicine is significant.

Bulimia nervous disorders, anorexia nervosa, and binge eating are characterized by unhealthy eating habits, which may include either insufficient or excessive consumption of food. They can eventually lead to severe physical or mental illnesses and diseases. Fasting can have severe consequences for a person with one of these disorders. People with an eating disorder who end up fasting may try to catch up on all of the food they have abstained from, in only a few days during the fast. This experience could enhance your eating disorder considerably.

The overall health of someone who wishes to follow this program should be evaluated before fasting. Fasting only for a few days is seldom a problem. However, if you have previously followed a junk food diet, it can cause problems. Also, if you have severe issues with your kidneys or liver or potential issues with your immune system or medications, then you should not try to start the fasting method.

The length of the first fast should not be stressful. If you don't think that you can last more than two days, don't push yourself. You can try doing it for three days the following week, and so on. This will acclimatize your body and brain to this new experience. You can also try to fast with drinking liquids for some days or distilled water. Some people start fasting at the age of 25 for 19 days, but not everyone can do that; you can start whenever you feel ready to train your body. A little bit at a time.

You need a passion for achieving your goals A quick way of achieving your goal or vision is to stay motivated. My motivation for fasting was to remove my body from a severe condition. This was the worst-case my doctor ever saw for someone as young as me. He said that the 1000 mg Zyloprim he prescribed would eventually destroy my kidneys.

Fasting to detoxify the body cannot get rid of toxins when your body is undernourished from the proper nutrients. The fact of the matter is that over 50% of American diets include processed fast foods, so people do not get the right amount of antioxidants and phytochemicals that help to protect our cells against damage. The cellular toxins produced lead to the destruction, aging, atherosclerosis, nerve diabetes, and organ loss, these conditions that are taught in all medical schools can be fixed with fasting since it is a proven healthy diet and the solution to remove AGE from cell tissues effectively.

When you follow distilled water fasting for more than a few days, the body runs out of carbohydrates to burn energy and cause ketosis. Your organism must burn fat in this case, and the fat is where the body retains chemicals and toxins that are ingested from the atmosphere and foods that we consume.

Fasting is even followed for medical surgeries. The patient must fast before the procedure to avoid complications when the body tries to digest food under anesthesia. Specific therapeutic procedures for cholesterol, various and blood sugar laboratory tests are also required to help and get accurate results.

Fasting when you are suffering from arthritis, lupus, skin disorders such as eczema and psoriasis has been shown to eliminate those. Distilled fasting with water also cured digestive conditions like ulcerative colitis and Crohn's disease. Even low blood pressure was treated with fasting successfully.

The studies of the National Academy of Sciences and The Journal of Nutrition show fasting mice achieved better insulin control, neuronal resistance, and several other health benefits over calorie-controlled mice when those were forced to fast every other day. On the non-fast day, scientists gave to the mice the reasonable food portion twice. Psychological benefits of fasting deal with stress and depression by straightening chemical imbalances in the body.

Not all weight loss diets are good for one's health and wellbeing. Some may prescribe lifestyle and dietary changes that can disrupt the natural balance of hormones, chemicals, and processes in your body. No matter what those changes are, the common goal among them is calorie deficit.

Other forms of diet may work for you for a given period of time because they encourage calorie restriction through various means. What sets apart fasting from those diets is the fact that it is, by far, the healthiest, fastest, and safest way to control your calorie intake.

Reducing the amount of calories in your diet is an essential component of any healthy and effective weight loss strategy. The great thing about fasting is that you do not have to worry about keeping count of the calories you are getting from your meals and drinks. Simply by skipping some meals or an entire day's worth of meals will decrease your caloric intake.

Just keep in mind, however, that fasting will not compensate for poor dietary choices. To get the most out of its weight loss effects, you should combine with a balanced diet, and regular exercise.

There is no standard amount of weight that people can lose through fasting. The actual amount varies greatly from one person to the other.

In general, those who have been obese for a long period of time would need to be more patient with the outcomes of their efforts to go through fasting.

There are also certain medications, including insulin, that could hamper your progress in losing weight. In such cases, all you can do is continue being persistent and patient with the method and with yourself.

At a certain point, you may also experience a plateau in the amount of weight you are losing through fasting. This means that you are no longer losing weight because the amount you lose when you were in a fasted state is equal to the amount of weight you gain whenever you eat again.

Avoiding this completely would require you to continue to fast for several weeks or months at a time. However, that is not possible for everyone, especially those who could only commit to controlled fasts.

The best way you can do to get over this plateau is changing your diet and/or regimen. For example, some people choose to extend their intermittent fasting periods from 24 hours to 36 hours. There are also individuals who can push themselves and go for a full 48-hour fast. Those who are following the Fast diet can simply lessen their meals from two to one per day, every day for a given week. You are free to think of other ways to get over the weight-loss plateau. Just switch things up, and observe if you will begin losing weight again from your fast.

Experts have also noted that there is a period of rapid weight loss during the early stages of fasting. Take note that this is not due to the loss of body fat, but rather just your excess water weight.

On an average, weight loss due to the burning of fat stores in your body has a rate of around 0.5 pounds per day. If you have noticed that you are losing more than 1 pound of body weight per day, then anything in excess of 0.5 pounds is likely just water weight.

The thing is, water weight can easily be regained when you feed again. Therefore, you should not be frustrated or disappointed when the large amount of body weight you have lost returns at some point during your fast.

This does not mean that fasting is not working for you. You are simply keeping track of something that is not accurately depicting the actual progress you are making during your fast.

To help you get a better idea of well you are doing during your fast, the next chapter shall tackle the various means available nowadays to effectively track your progress.

Chapter 7 – How to Track Progress While Fasting

As with any lifestyle plan and diet, the best way to start tracking your progress is by keeping a benchmark of key determining variables, such as weighing yourself regularly, monitoring body fat levels, and going through routine blood tests.

Such measures are necessary to get an objective reflection of the progress that you have made so far during your fast. If you are not aware of the condition your body was in when you first started, then it is hard to appreciate the positive effects of fasting on your body.

People who fail to recognize their importance tend to run the risk of losing their motivation to push through the low moments of fasting. Furthermore, knowing exactly where you are standing would also keep you from straying away from your goals.

For your guidance, here are the common methods used to gauge progress while engaging in a fast:

- Body Mass Index (BMI) Monitoring

Rather than simply relying on your body weight alone, you should calculate for your body mass index instead. This refers to the ratio of your weight and height. By computing for this, you would be able to tell whether you are still in the normal weight range for a person of your size, or if you have already become underweight or overweight.

You may determine your BMI by following these steps:

1. Measure your body weight and height.

   o If you have taken your weight in pounds, you should convert it to kilograms by following this formula:

   Weight in Pounds ÷ 2.2 = Weight in Kilograms

   For example:

   110 pounds ÷ 2.2 = 50 kilograms

   o If you have measured your height in inches, convert it to meters by using this formula:

   Height in Inches ÷ 39.37 = Height in Meters

   For example:

   60 inches ÷ 39.37 = 1.52 meters

2. Divide your body weight by the product of your height multiplied by itself, as demonstrated by the example below:

   Weight in Kilograms ÷ (Height in Meters x Height in Meters) = Body Mass Index

   50 kilograms ÷ (1.52 meters x 1.52 meters) = 21.64

3. Refer to the standard BMI ranges to determine your weight status.

   o Below 18.50 = Underweight
   o Between 18.50 and 24.90 = Normal Weight
   o Between 25.00 and 29.90 = Overweight
   o 30.00 and above = Obese

For faster computation, you may also consider using an online BMI calculator, or downloading a BMI app in your phone. Based on the example given above, a person with a height of 60 inches and a weight of 110 pounds is still within the normal range.

Focusing solely on your weight as an indicator of your progress is not recommended. No matter how accurate your bathroom scale is, it cannot tell you what your fat-to-muscle ratio is.

It can also mislead you to believe that you are not making progress at all. Some people have noticed that their body weights have gone up after they have started living healthier and more active lifestyles. At first glance, it may seem that the changes they have made only worsened their condition. However, lean muscle mass weighs more than body fat, thus making you physically denser the more you develop your muscles.

BMI will not show your exact body composition at a given moment. It is, however, one of the simplest and least expensive ways of monitoring the amount of weight you have lost since you have begun fasting.

Body Fat Testing

To determine your body composition, many fitness experts recommend undergoing body fat testing. This may be done through body composition scales, body fat calipers, and water/air displacement test.

o   Body Composition Scales

This equipment promises to measure the overall body-fat ratio through a wide, but inconsistent scope of variables, such as body hydration, and feet condition. As such, you should take the measurements from body composition scales with a grain of salt.

According to a recent study, this equipment tends to overestimate the body fat of leaner individuals, such as healthy adults and athletes. On the other hand, these scales underestimate the amount of body fat that overweight and obese people have.

Some manufacturers have tried to address these findings by developing handheld body composition scales that are designed to provide more accurate readings. Further studies show that the improvements are only marginal at best.

o Body Fat Calipers

This method should be done with the assistance of a medical professional or a physical trainer who has experience in using calipers to measure your body fat.

The equipment works by pinching the fat on various areas of your body, such as the triceps, navel, and hips. The measurements obtained from the calipers are then inputted into an equation that can determine your body fat percentage.

The major disadvantage with this method is the probability of your physician or trainer committing an error during the actual measurements itself. As a result, you may be given inaccurate figures about your body fat.

o Water/Air Displacement Test

This is considered as one of the most accurate ways to determine your body composition. The principle behind these tests is based on the original concept of Archimedes, an ancient Greek philosopher, about volume and density.

In general, both tests require the usage of highly precise weight scales, and specialized equipment that can determine your volume. As such, these tests tend to be costly. A single test normally costs around $50.00.

Routine Blood Tests

Ideally, you should undergo a routine blood test before going into a fast, and after 90 days since you have started fasting. The great thing about these tests is that they are usually inexpensive, and it may even be covered by your health insurance.

A regular routine blood test may include the following checkpoints:

Cholesterol Levels

Results under this checkpoint are categorized into two: HDL and LDL.

High-Density Lipoprotein (HDL) refers to the good cholesterol in your bloodstream, whose main purpose is to eliminate bad cholesterol from your system. High amounts of HDL is a good sign for your cardiovascular health as well.

On the other hand, Low-Density Lipoprotein (LDL) pertains to the bad cholesterol that tends to accumulate on the walls of your blood vessels. Having high levels of LDL indicates that you are at risk of developing certain forms of heart diseases and stroke.

What you want to see from your results is a good ratio in favor of HDL rather than LDL.

Fasting can help you obtain such results, along with a diet that is rich in healthy fats, such as avocados and walnuts. Eating less processed foods—like energy bars, pre-packed meals, and breakfast cereals—and food products that are high in trans-fat—such as potato chips, cakes, and donuts—will help you decrease your LDL levels.

Triglycerides

When you burn less fat than what you have consumed, the triglycerides found in your blood become part of your stored body fat. At most, you should only have 100 milligrams of triglycerides per 1 deciliter of your blood. Higher amounts of triglycerides can increase your risk of developing cardiovascular diseases.

Fasting Blood Glucose

> This test is used to measure the amount of glucose in your blood after you have abstained from food for eight hours. Blood glucose tends to rise up after eating. However, if it remains on an elevated level even after going through a brief fasting period, then you are either diabetic, or at a high risk of becoming diabetic.

> When this condition continues to persist for a long period of time, key areas of your body, such as the pancreas, eyes, and kidneys, would become damaged.

Regardless of which method you end up choosing, make it a point to record every measurement in a journal or logbook. Normally, you would be seeing a downward trend of your body fat from the moment you have started fasting.

However, do not dwell on these numbers, especially when they are not meeting your expectations. Remember, this is only one aspect of your journey towards attaining a healthier and longer life.

Tracking Your Progress through Mobile Apps

Nowadays, you can find an app for almost anything you want. Using a mobile app to track your progress is not only a convenient way to record your experiences, but also a cheap way to get a comprehensive visual report on the changes that have happened in your body since you have started fasting.

Here are a couple of apps that you should try in order to effectively track your progress.

- Zero

    Use this app if your fasting schedule is consistent day after day. To start, you must identify first your fasting regimen from the list indicated in the app. This includes popular choices such as 16:8 intermittent fasting and the circadian rhythm option, wherein your fast lasts from sunset up to the following morning. If your fasting regimen is not included in the list, then you may customize the schedule for up to a 7-day period.

    Based on your preferred daily fasting strategy, the app would track the number of hours you have fasted for the past seven days, and how much weight you have lost during that period. It can also send you notifications whenever your fasting period is about to start or end.

    As an added value for its users, links to research studies, podcasts, and videos about fasting are provided in the app as well.

    Availability: iOS, Android

Cost: Free

- LIFE Fasting Tracker

  If you prefer fasting in a group setting, then this app would allow you to share your progress with your family, friends, and other important people in your life. Through this, you may also issue challenges to your social groups, and keep each other accountable of your commitment to fast.

  You may use this if you are engaging in any time-restricted fasting schedule, such as the One-Meal-A-Day method, or 16:8 intermittent fasting. Aside from tracking your weight, the app may also be used to record the measurements of your waistline, glucose levels, and the ketones in your system.

  This app also provides its users new research articles about fasting on a weekly basis.

  Availability: iOS, Android

  Cost: Free

Chapter 8 – How to Ward off the Potential Negative Effects from Fasting

You might feel the negative effects of fasting due to any combination of these three factors: hunger, lack of motivation, and low energy levels. To prevent you from suffering, here are the top strategies you can employ to combat these three factors.

Top 10 Ways to Keep Hunger at Bay While Fasting

Hunger itself does not make fasting difficult for you. It is your reaction towards it that makes things more complicated during fasting. Normally, when you feel hunger, you would appease it by eating food. When you cannot get over that reaction, then you do not have control over hunger—rather, it is controlling you.

It is hard to just ignore your hunger pangs when you are just sitting around throughout your fast. Therefore, you must learn how to keep hunger at bay while staying active and productive during your fasting period.

Here are the top 10 strategies that you can do to achieve such goals.

1. Accept that hunger is a natural aspect of fasting.

   You can only start controlling hunger when you accept it for what it is—a natural reaction of your body to the absence of food.

   Many anthropologists even suggest that the human body should naturally be in a hungry state for most of the day, while well-fed and well-rested by nighttime.

   Therefore, sustaining the balance between feeding and fasting is essential in attaining good health.

2. Drink lots of water.

   Studies show that the simplest and healthiest way to reduce the intensity and frequency of hunger pangs is through the consumption of adequate amounts of water throughout the day.

   More often than not, people tend to mistake their thirst for hunger. Drinking more water rather than eating a snack is the right approach to deal with your hunger while fasting.

   Aside from the amount of water you are drinking, you should also be mindful of its quality. Make sure that your drinking water is free from toxins, hormones, and other harmful chemicals.

3. Drink a nice cup of coffee or tea.

   The caffeine in these beverages may suppress feelings of hunger when consumed in moderation.

   Because coffee has higher caffeine content, it is more effective than any kind of tea there is. However, be careful not to drink it after noon has already passed. Otherwise, you would have trouble sleeping later on.

4. Snack on raw foods.

   If you simply cannot go through a fasting period without eating anything, then you might want to consider engaging in a controlled fast instead. This is the same principle applied to the undereating phase of the Warrior Diet.

   During a controlled fast, you would be allowed to eat foods that would not be difficult to digest, and would not significantly increase your blood sugar levels.

   Therefore, the best kinds of food that you can eat are raw fruits and vegetables that have low glycemic index. Examples of such foods include strawberries, raspberries, blueberries, carrots, broccoli, and ginger. Be careful not to overeat them, however. The ideal serving size is only a handful of these fruits and vegetables.

5. Go for a walk.

    Walking briskly while you are in the middle of a fast enhances the fat-burning processes going on inside your body. It would also serve as your cardio workout for that given day, thus contributing to your efforts in keeping your heart in tip-top condition.

    Like most forms of exercises, walking can suppress your hunger. However, the great thing about it is that it does not require as much energy from you as the other more intense physical activities.

6. Play recreational sports.

    Any recreational sports, such as basketball, swimming, or tennis, can enhance the positive effects of fasting on your health. As an added bonus, you would be able to trick your mind away from focusing on the signals sent by your empty stomach.

7. Do some household chores.

    These are positive distractions from hunger pangs. Your focus will be on other things that could also benefit not just you, but also the people you live with.

You may clean different areas of the house, or go out and do some gardening. But, basically, anything that could keep you occupied during your fasted state may be an effective means of keeping the hunger at bay.

8. Accomplish some work-related tasks.

Similarly, you may also distract yourself by finishing off your pending tasks from work.

Many people even find it meditative to answer to emails, and clean up the inbox during such days. You may also try finishing a report that you need to submit soon.

Again, keep in mind that the busier you are, the easier it would be for you to push through the fast.

9. Make time for your hobbies.

Recent studies show that non-physical hobbies can have similar effects as physical activities when it comes to distracting yourself from hunger. Just make sure that they are mentally stimulating for you. Examples of such hobbies include reading, playing a musical instrument, or creating artworks.

10. Meditate.

Through meditation, you would be able to exert more control over your thoughts and feelings. It may not be the easiest way to suppress your hunger, especially if you are not an experienced meditator (read PRACTICAL MEDITATIONS FOR BEGINNERS by RAQUEL PEG - ISBN-978-1705692332). However, over time and regular practice, this may be the most effective means of keeping your hunger at bay while fasting.

Top 10 Ways to Stay Motivated While Fasting

Some people who undergo fasting may experience low mood, insecurities, and anxiety during the course of their fast. Aside from the general lack of food, this mostly stems from all the adjustment they have to make in their life, and the frustration over their progress towards their fitness goals.

You may combat such negative effects by keeping your motivation up despite the challenges that you are experiencing during your fast. Here are the top motivational tactics that you may try doing. Feel free to combine and use any of these tactics to figure out which ones would best work for you.

1. Enlist the help of someone who can keep you accountable.

Select a family member, a friend, or even a co-worker who can keep you on track and motivate you throughout your fasting period. Getting their support would help you in avoiding temptations, and giving in to your doubts and insecurities.

If there is no one near who could fit the bill, you may turn to social media and fasting apps that enable users to connect with one another, even if you live across the world from them.

2. Watch motivational videos, or read inspiring articles and blog posts.

Many people find it helpful to see, hear, or read about the success stories of other individuals who have gone through fasting. Doing so would help you visualize the future that you want for yourself, too.

Just make sure that the material that you are viewing or listening to would motivate you for the right reasons. The right material would inspire you to reach for your goals, not make you feel bad for not making similar strides as other people do.

3. Establish short-term goals with a tempting reward. Rather simply focusing on your end goal for fasting, you should try creating measurable goals that you may attain in a day or two. Though many people who are engaging in fasting think that food is the

best reward for such accomplishments, try to refrain from doing so. Instead, opt for healthier options, such as getting yourself a massage, or purchasing a new set of workout clothes.

Making food as your reward would only increase your feelings of deprivation during your fast. Therefore, it would be self-sabotaging to the progress that you have made so far.

4. Set personal punishments for not meeting your goals.

A good, but tricky way to ensure that you are on track is by deciding what you would do in case you fail to achieve your goals. Some people make their least preferred household chore as their punishment, while others think that simply not getting the supposed reward is enough punishment for them.

Keep in mind, however, that making extended food deprivation periods as your punishment is not recommended. The same goes for punishing yourself by having to do extra rounds of exercising. Doing so would condition your mind against these healthy practices, thereby making it harder for you to fully commit to a healthy and active lifestyle.

5. Imagine your future state if you would quit fasting now.

   Close your eyes, and visualize your answers to these questions:

   o If you were to quit now, what would your appearance be like in a couple of months? What would be your health condition?

   o If you were to revert back to your unhealthy practices, how much weight would you gain in a couple of months?

   o Will you feel ashamed of your decision to quit fasting? Why or why not?

   Be honest with yourself and think hard about your future with and without fasting. By doing so, you would be able to better appreciate the effects of fasting on your health and overall quality of life.

6. Visualize your desired future.

   The future is uncertain, and therefore, many find it scary. Imagining what you want to achieve is one way of dissipating the fog that may be surrounding your mind. Through visualization, you would also learn the aspects of your life that must be changed or controlled in order to attain that future.

   Try not to dwell on your negative thoughts and insecurities during this mental exercise. If they do enter your mind while you are in the middle of your visualizations, take a pause, breathe, and realign your focus on the positive side of things.

7. Focus on your positive emotions.

If you are having a hard time in staying positive, recall moments in your life where you felt happy or accomplished while embracing your new lifestyle. It may be when you managed to resist the temptation of going for another cup of coffee, or the time you received a compliment from your co-workers about your more refreshed look.

Remembering and reliving these positive moments would bring out the positive emotions out of you. Moreover, when you are feeling positive, it is easier to stay motivated despite the challenges that you may be facing at the moment.

8. Re-evaluate your goals.

If you are feeling demotivated because you do not think you are making enough progress, then you might need to check how well you have crafted your goals. Perhaps they are not specific and measurable, thus making it hard for you to recognize the progress you have made. It may be even constructed in a way that would prevent you from determining whether or not you have actually achieved your goals.

Take the time to re-evaluate the quality of your goals, and if needed, feel free to adjust them according to your current status and desires. It is your personal goal, so you have complete control over them.

9. Be kinder to yourself.

Whenever you encounter setbacks while you are fasting, the best thing you can do is being compassionate to your own self. Do not engage in negative self-talk if you are not meeting your targets.

Instead, assess the situation you are in, and figure out how you can do better from then on. By doing so, you would be able to turn your low moments into something more constructive and productive.

10. Form a habit of motivating yourself.

Set aside at least 15 minutes per day to think about your goals, and what you have accomplished so far. Then, recite to yourself some positive affirmations that can motivate you to keep going on.

Here are some examples of positive affirmations that you can try for yourself:

o "I am so thankful for my good health, and supportive family and friends."

o "I want to live a long, happy, and healthy life with my loved ones."

o "My health is one of my greatest assets, and I invest in that asset through my daily thoughts and actions."

o "I am strong, patient, and compassionate."

You can practice this exercise in front of a mirror, in the car, or whenever you are alone. You are also not required to do this all in one go. Break it into several 3 to 5-minute sessions throughout the day, if that would be more convenient for you. Just make time for this activity every day so that it would gradually become a normal part of your daily routine.

Top 10 Ways to Remain Energetic While Fasting

A common assumption among most people is that you can only get energy from the foods you are eating. However, studies show that eating can actually make you feel less energized because the influx of insulin released after you have taken your meal is used to aid the digestion of the food you have eaten. As a result, many people feel the urge to take a nap after having a big meal.

On the other hand, you might feel less energetic during the initial stages of fasting. However, there are various means to effectively raise your energy levels even while you are in a fasted state. Here are the top 10 ways that you can employ to combat the negative effects of fasting on your energy levels.

1. Stand up and move around.

   More often than not, those who feel sluggish during a fast blame their condition on the lack of food. However, studies show that a sedentary lifestyle can be detrimental for sustaining optimal blood flow and energy levels.

   Therefore, to feel more energized, you should try getting up from your seat, and go for a walk. You may also stretch out your limbs, or even perform brief workout sessions.

   You may be too immersed with whatever you are doing at the time, so remind yourself by setting up an alarm every hour.

2. Play a casual game.

   Games can help boost your energy while decreasing your stress levels at the same time. For this to be a more effective strategy, you should set a time limit whenever you are going to play a game. This would keep you from becoming too engrossed in it that you would neglect your other activities for the day.

3. Socialize more with the people around you.

   Interacting with other people has plenty of benefits when it comes to keeping you in your best condition while fasting. It can serve as an excellent distraction from the physical and mental strain of fasting, thus keeping you from succumbing to hunger and stress.

   Furthermore, if you choose to socialize with people who are supportive of your decision to fast, then you would feel more refreshed and energized after having a chat with them.

4. Smile and laugh more.

   A simple smile can improve your mood, and make you feel less weary. Moreover, laughing stimulates both the body and mind, while giving your energy levels a nice boost.

   Research shows that most adults laugh only five times a day, while children have an average of 300 times per day. You can emulate the energetic and optimistic outlook of young children by finding things in your life that you smile or laugh about.

5. Drink plenty of water.

Dehydration is one of the major, but frequently overlooked causes of fatigue. Even if you are only experiencing mild dehydration, your body would find it hard to perform several critical functions, such as nutrient transportation, and waste removal.

To keep you from dehydration while you are fasting, drink more than the recommended amount per day. Aim to drink 10 to 12 glasses of water throughout the day. By doing so, you would be able to keep your energy high even while you are consuming less food than you usually do.

6. Get an energy boost from caffeine.

Studies show that the right amount of caffeine can be beneficial to keeping your energy up during a fast. It can also help you concentrate better on your physical and mental activities.

Drinking more caffeine, however, is not recommended since it will negatively affect the quality and schedule of your sleep. Healthy caffeinated beverages, such as coffee and tea, should be consumed during the earlier parts of the day. Also, limit yourself to a maximum of two cups per day. Following these suggestions would prevent caffeine from interfering with your normal sleep routine.

7. Engage in energizing aromatherapy.

    Here are some of the highly recommended scents that can boost your energy, even when you are not fasting:

o   Citrus

    Effects: Improves level of concentration

o   Lavender

    Effects: Calms the mind, and brightens up the mood

o   Rosemary

    Effects: Sharpens the alertness of the mind, and increases memory retention

    Through aromatherapy, you may be able to improve your productivity, and increase your brain activity. You only need to inhale a few drops of these scents using a scent diffuser or even just on a cotton ball. For optimal results, do this activity in the morning, or whenever you need a little boost throughout the day.

8. Listen to your favorite music.

    Research shows that listening to music promotes better blood flow to the brain, thereby stimulating your mind in the process. Certain kinds of music have also been observed to cause various effects to the body and mind. For instance, classical music can energize you, while most pop music can turn away your focus from whatever you are doing.

To boost your energy through music, grab your headphones, and take the time to listen intently. Better yet, make a playlist of your favorite songs so that you can easily play something that you would quickly find something pleasant to listen to.

9. Have a more active sex life.

    Engaging in sex increases the production and release of endorphins—or the brain chemical that can make you feel better and more energized. Doing it more frequently could then help stabilize your energy levels even when you are not getting the same amount of food that you used to.

10. Get enough high-quality sleep.

    To keep yourself from feeling exhausted, you should always try to get a good night's sleep. Here are some tips on how you can improve the quality of your sleep:

○   Create and stick to a sleep routine.

○   Avoid drinking caffeinated drinks too late in the day or in the evening.

○   Do not rely on alcoholic drinks to make you fall asleep.

o   Turn off all electronic devices, like your
    cellphone or tablet, at least one hour before
    going to bed.

o   If you are sleeping during daytime, install
    blackout curtains to prevent natural light
    from streaming into your bedroom.

o   Maintain an optimal, ambient temperature
    in your bedroom.

Chapter 9 – Sample Kick-Start Fasting Plan and Some Recipes That You Should Try

Committing to a fasting plan can be quite daunting for beginners. There are many unknown variables that can chip away at your self-confidence. You might think that you would not be able to handle the hunger pangs well enough to successfully go through the full fasting period. Someone else's experience during fasting might discourage you from pursuing your fasting goals. In some cases, the people around you might actively dissuade you from fasting due to their incorrect assumptions about your capability or the practice itself.

Whichever the case may be, you should keep in mind that you do not have to dive in with both feet, and simply hope for the best. Beginners can kick-start their fasting through gradual, but even steps that are easy to follow.

To demonstrate how this is possible, here is a detailed fasting plan that you may implement for a period of 7 to 10 days, depending on how much time you need to kick-start your fasting. Recipes for selected menu items are also given below so that you could try recreating them in your own kitchen.

You should also keep a journal, and jot down your thoughts and observations for each day. This would serve as a valuable reference for you later on when you have gone through this kick-start plan.

Day 1

Your objective for the first day of your kick-start plan is to avoid consuming anything after you have had your dinner.

Since you are not yet used to this, try doing these simple tips on how to get through the night without snacking after dinner.

o   Rather than eating food as snacks, you should have a warm cup of relaxing herbal tea instead. In case you are not fond of tea, a glass of water could be a healthier substitute as well.

o   Brush your teeth after eating your dinner. Normally, you would brush your teeth at night when you are done eating for the day. Therefore, the minty taste of your toothpaste could help condition your brain against giving in to your cravings.

- Go to bed earlier. This would prevent you from feeling the urge to go snacking after dinner.

Here is the suggested meal plan for this day:

- Breakfast
    - Apple Berry Smoothie*
- Morning Snack
    - Any fruit in season
- Lunch
    - Taco Salad with Guacamole
- Afternoon Snack
    - Unsalted Mixed Nuts
- Dinner
    - Broccoli Mushroom Bisque

If you want to try making the Apple Berry Smoothie, here is its recipe:

Ingredients

- 1 apple, core removed
- 1 cucumber, small-sized only
- 1 cup strawberries
- ½ cup milk (soy, hemp, or almond), unsweetened
- 2 tablespoons rolled oats

- 1 tablespoon ground chia seeds
- 1 tablespoon Mediterranean pine nuts
- 1 teaspoon cinnamon

Directions

1. Place all ingredients into a high-powered blender.

2. Mix all ingredients until texture has become smooth.

3. Pour into your preferred containers.

4. Consume immediately.

Yield

Makes 2 servings

Day 2

For Day 2 of the kick-start plan, your objective is to postpone your breakfast, and skip your morning snack.

Since you have not consumed anything since your dinner from the night before, you have already undergone around 12 hours of fasting. That is excellent because technically, you have been on a fasted state for half a day already. It was also not hard on you because you were asleep for the most part of it.

Now, your goal is to extend that fasting period to 15 hours. You can drink water, unsweetened coffee, or tea in the morning, but avoid consuming any kind of breakfast food or morning snack.

By doing so, you would be building on to what you have started during your first day. You should also continue your practice of having no snacks after eating your dinner.

Here is the recommended menu for Day 2 of your kick-start plan:

- o Lunch
    - ▪ Slow-Cooked Eggplant*
- o Afternoon Snack
    - ▪ Any fruit in season
- o Dinner
    - ▪ Three Bean Mango Salad

Make advanced preparations for your lunch during this day by following this recipe for Slow-Cooked Eggplant.

Ingredients

- 1 eggplant, cut into ½ inch cubes
- 1 apple, core removed, and chopped
- 2 cups tomato, chopped
- 6 ounces tomato paste

- 1 ½ cups chickpeas
- 1 ½ cups carrot juice
- 1 ½ cups vegetable broth, unsalted
- 1 cup white onion, chopped
- 1 teaspoon cinnamon
- ½ teaspoon nutmeg

Directions

1. Place the eggplant, apple, tomatoes, chickpeas, and onion into a crockpot.

2. Combine the tomato paste, carrot juice, vegetable broth, cinnamon, and nutmeg in a separate bowl.

3. Pour the mixture over the vegetables and fruits inside the crockpot.

4. Cover the crockpot with its lid.

5. Cook on low heat for 7 to 8 hours.

6. Turn off the crockpot to cool down its contents.

7. Serve, and consume immediately.

Yield

Makes 4 servings

Day 3

Your main goal for Day 3 is to reduce your calorie intake. To do so, you must delay your breakfast, and skip both your morning snack and afternoon snack.

Many people find it necessary to eat snacks in the afternoon, especially since this period tends to be the busiest. However, your afternoon snack is keeping you from losing weight faster.

Here are some effective but simple tips that can condition your body and mind against taking your afternoon snack.

o Remind yourself that dinnertime is only a couple of hours away. At this point, all you have to do is wait for the right timing to eat.

o In most cases, the hunger you are feeling in the afternoon is not actually hunger. You might only be thirsty, or you might be feeling stressed out, bored, or anxious. Rather than giving in to the urge to eat something, drink a glass of water, a cup of black coffee, or a cup of herbal tea instead.

For Day 3, here is the suggested meal plan that you should follow:

o Breakfast

  ▪ Breakfast Bars*

- o Lunch
  - Stuffed Bell Peppers
- o Dinner
  - Creamy Zucchini Soup

Making the Breakfast Bars at home is simple and easy, as illustrated by its recipe below.

Ingredients

- 1 cup old-fashion oats
- 1 ripe banana
- 1 cup frozen blueberries, thawed out
- 1 cup cooked black beans, low-salt or unsalted
- ½ cup California raisins
- ½ cup pomegranate juice
- 2 tablespoons ground flax seed
- 2 tablespoons dates, finely chopped
- 2 tablespoons sunflower seeds
- 2 tablespoons goji berries
- 1 tablespoon walnuts, chopped
- extra-virgin olive oil (for greasing the baking pan only)

Directions

1. Pre-heat the oven to 275 °F (135 °C).

2. Puree the black beans in a high-powered blender or food processor.

3. Mash the banana in a bowl.

4. Add the pureed black beans and the rest of the ingredients into the bowl.

5. Mix well the ingredients.

6. Brush lightly an 8-inch baking pan with extra-virgin olive oil.

7. Spread the mixture on the baking pan.

8. Bake in the oven for 75 minutes.

9. Cool down the baked goods on a wire rack.

10. Slice into 2-inch by 2-inch bars.

11. Consume immediately, or store in the refrigerator for up to 3 days.

Yield

Makes 6 servings

Day 4

For your fourth day into the kick-start plan, your aim is to extend your fasting duration by skipping your breakfast, morning snack, and sustaining your reduced calorie intake by not taking your afternoon snack as well.

By doing this, your first meal for the day would be during lunch time already. Make sure to continue your good practice of abstaining from food right away after dinner.

Here is the suggested menu for Day 4 of the kick-start plan.

- o Lunch

    - ▪ Homemade Baked Chicken Fingers*

- o Dinner

    - ▪ Arugula and Pear Salad

Going into a fast does not mean that you are completely forbidden from enjoying crispy and crunchy dishes. You just have to cook them in ways that would eliminate the harmful toxins associated with frying. For example, try out this recipe for Homemade Baked Chicken Fingers—a healthier option in case you are craving for fried chicken.

Ingredients

- • 1 pound boneless chicken breast, cut into 1-inch x 3-inch strips
- • 2 eggs
- • 1 cup pork cracklings, crushed
- • 2 tablespoons coconut oil
- • 1 tablespoon salt
- • 1 teaspoon garlic salt (optional)
- • 1 teaspoon ground black pepper
- • 1 teaspoon smoked paprika

Directions

1. Pre-heat the oven to 300 °F (148.89 °C).

2. Line a baking tray with aluminum foil.

3. Pat dry the washed chicken strips.

4. Combine the crushed pork cracklings, salt, garlic salt (if you are using), black pepper, and paprika in a small bowl.

5. Pour the dry mixture into a re-sealable plastic bag.

6. Beat the eggs in a medium-sized bowl.

7. Coat each chicken strip with beaten egg.

8. Place the coated chicken strip into the re-sealable plastic bag with the dry mixture.

9. Seal well before shaking the bag to evenly coat the chicken strips.

10. Arrange the chicken fingers into the baking tray.

11. Bake in the oven for about 10 to 15 minutes.

12. Flip over the chicken fingers.

13. Bake for another 10 to 15 minutes, or until the chicken fingers are golden brown.

14. Remove the chicken fingers from the oven.

15. Let them cool for about 5 minutes.

16. Consume immediately.

Yield

Makes 2 servings

Day 5

Your goal for Day 5 is to sustain the fasting period and eating practices that you had done the previous day. This would help you maintain the momentum that fasting has gained so far.

For your reference, here is a meal plan that would enable you to skip breakfast and snacking without feeling the negative side-effects of fasting.

- Lunch
    - Roasted Cauliflower Rice*
    - Salmon Fillet with Lemon Glaze
- Dinner
    - Avocado, Tomato, and Cucumber Salad

Loading up on carbohydrates at this point is not recommended. Fortunately, the Roasted Cauliflower Rice can trick your brain into thinking that you are eating rice along with your salmon during lunch. Here is a simple recipe that even beginners can follow without fail.

Ingredients

- 1 head cauliflower
- ½ tablespoon salt
- Spices and herbs (optional)

Directions

1. Pre-heat the oven to 200 °F (93.33 °C).

2. Line a baking tray with parchment paper.

3. Chop the cauliflower into florets.

4. Remove the stem from each cauliflower floret.

5. Grate the cauliflower using a manual grater or food processor until its appearance becomes similar to rice grains.

6. Arrange the cauliflower rice on the baking tray.

7. Sprinkle salt evenly on the cauliflower rice.

8. Place the baking tray inside the oven

9. Bake for 12 to 15 minutes, flipping and stirring every few minutes.

10. Remove the cauliflower rice from the oven before it turns brown.

11. Season with spices or herbs, if desired.

12. Consume immediately.

Yield

Makes 2 servings

If you want to extend further your kick-start period, then continue following the fasting plan for Days 6 and 7.

Day 6

Day 6 of the kick-start plan is to lengthen the duration of your fasting period by around 3 to 4 hours. This can be achieved by skipping your breakfast, morning snack, and lunch, thus making your afternoon snack your first meal of the day.

As such, it is important for your selection of an afternoon snack to be filling yet healthy. Here is the suggested menu that can get you through your sixth day into the kick-start plan.

- o Afternoon Snack

  - ▪ Chia Seed Cookies*

- o Dinner

- Baked Tofu with Mushroom Wine Sauce

You can keep a stock of Chia Seed Cookies as your go-to snack during the earlier parts of the kick-start plan. To bake them on your own, here is an easy recipe that you can follow:

Ingredients

- 2 cups rolled oats, finely ground
- 1 cup currants
- ¾ cup apple sauce, unsweetened
- ½ cup dried coconut, shredded and unsweetened
- 2 tablespoons almond butter, raw
- 1 tablespoon whole chia seeds
- 1 tablespoon ground chia seeds
- 1 teaspoon vanilla
- 1 teaspoon cinnamon

Directions

1. Pre-heat the oven to 200 °F (93.33 °C).

2. Soak half of the currants in ½ cup of water for at least 60 minutes.

3. Combine the ground rolled oats, shredded coconut, whole and ground chia seeds, cinnamon, and the remaining currants in a bowl.

4. Put the soaked currants and the soaking water, applesauce, almond butter, and vanilla in a food processor.

5. Blend the ingredients until the texture has become smooth.

6. Add the dry ingredients into the contents of the mixture.

7. Stir well.

8. Create cookies from 2 teaspoons of dough for each cookie.

9. Place the cookies on a lightly greased baking sheet.

10. Bake the cookies in the oven for 90 minutes up to 120 minutes, depending on your preference.

11. Remove the cookies from the oven.

12. Let the cookies cool down for 5 minutes.

13. Transfer into cookie containers for later consumption.

Yield

Makes 20 pieces

Day 7

By your seventh day, your body is ready to undergo a 4-hour window for your feeding time. As such, you would have to skip your breakfast, morning snack, lunch, and afternoon snack.

Your only meal for Day 7 of the kick-start plan is your dinner. Here is a good dish that you can try making for your dinner during this day: Zesty Brussels Sprouts with Walnuts.

Ingredients

- 1 pound Brussels sprouts
- ½ cup orange juice, freshly squeezed
- 1/3 cup walnuts, chopped
- 1 teaspoon grated orange zest
- A pinch of ground black pepper

Directions

1. Place Brussels sprouts in a steamer basket.

2. Place the steamer basket over a pot of boiling water.

3. Cover the steamer basket with its lid.

4. Steam for about 20 minutes, or until Brussels sprouts are tender.

5. Place the steamed Brussels sprouts and orange juice in a large pan.

6. Simmer for 3 minutes.

7. Remove from the heat.

8. Toast the walnuts in a separate skillet for about 2 to 3 minutes, or until walnuts are lightly toasted.

9. Add the toasted walnuts, grated orange zest into the Brussels sprouts.

10. Season with ground black pepper to taste.

11. Consume immediately.

Yield

Makes 4 servings

In case you feel like extending your kick-start plan even further, here is an additional 3-day plan that you can follow.

Day 8

Begin your extra days by keeping your goals from the previous day. You should eat your dinner only.

Mustard Green Beans is another dish that can give you the nutrients you would be needing to push through the following days. To prepare and cook it in the comforts of your own kitchen, here is a quick recipe for it:

Ingredients

- 1 pound green beans, trimmed
- 1 tablespoon mustard (any variant)
- 1 tablespoon extra-virgin olive oil
- A pinch of salt
- A pinch of ground black pepper

Directions

1. Fill a saucepan with water until it is three-quarters full.

2. Place a steam basket over the saucepan.

3. Bring the water to a boil using medium-high heat.

4. Place the green beans into the steamer basket.

5. Steam the green beans for about 5 minutes, or until they have become tender but still crispy.

6. Remove the beans from the steam basket.

7. In a non-stick skillet, heat the olive oil for about 5 minutes.

8. Stir in the mustard.

9. Add the steamed green beans into the mustard-oil mixture.

10. Cook for around 2 minutes, or until the contents of the pan are well mixed and heated through.

11. Remove the beans from the skillet.

12. Season with salt and pepper to taste.

13. Consume immediately.

Yield

Makes 4 servings

Day 9

Your objective for the ninth day into the kick-start plan is to incorporate simple cardio exercises into your routine. You still should only eat your dinner, even if you have to move around a bit more than usual.

Go out for a quick jog or perform brief aerobics exercises. Observe how your body would react from such activities. Normally, at this point, you should be feeling more energized after doing an exercise.

To replenish you, the suggested dinner for this is the Strawberry and Kale Salad. It is a simple dish to prepare that would only take you a matter of a few minutes to finish. Here is the recipe for this salad.

Ingredients

- 12 fresh strawberries, diced
- 4 cups fresh kale

- 1 cup walnuts, unsalted
- 4 tablespoons extra-virgin olive oil
- 1 tablespoon balsamic vinegar
- A pinch of salt
- A pinch of ground black pepper

Directions

1. Toss the strawberries, kale, and walnuts in a large bowl.

2. Pour the balsamic vinegar and olive oil all over the salad.

3. Season with salt and pepper.

4. Consume immediately.

Yield

Makes 2 servings

Day 10

Your ultimate goal for the kick-start plan is to go through a day by drinking fluids only. Some people assume that you can only drink water at this point, but experts do allow the consumption of certain drinks that would do well with the current condition of your body.

Also, remember that by the time you have reached Day 10, you have successfully gone through the kick-start plan for nine days. During that period, you have learned how to avoid eating out of habit, due to thirst, or as a way of improving your mood. Now, you only eat when you truly feel hunger.

As a guide, here is the recommended meal plan for the fluids-only day of the kick-start plan:

- o Breakfast
  - Water with Lemon Slices
- o Lunch
  - Bone Broth*
- o Dinner
  - Japanese Green Tea

As mentioned, earlier, you are not limited to only water. You are allowed to consume other types of healthy beverages, as well as homemade broth. Here is the recipe of the Bone Broth that you may have as your lunch for Day 10:

Ingredients

- 6 quarts cold water
- 2 pounds animal bones (beef, pork, poultry, or fish)
- 10 stalks celery, chopped
- 3 large carrots, chopped
- 1 medium red onion, chopped
- 1 green bell pepper, chopped
- 1 red bell pepper, chopped

- 2 tablespoons raw apple cider vinegar
- 1 tablespoon salt
- 1 tablespoon whole black peppercorns
- Other herbs and spices (optional, according to your taste preferences)

Directions

1. Pour 6 quarts of cold water into a stockpot.

2. Add the apple cider vinegar into the pot.

3. Place the animal bones inside the pot.

4. Add the chopped celery, carrots, onion, bell peppers, salt, pepper, dried herbs, and other spices (if you are using any) into the pot.

5. Place the pot over a stove in a medium-high heat setting.

6. Continue heating until the contents are nearly boiling.

7. Reduce the heat to low.

8. Simmer the broth according to the suggested duration for each type of animal bone:

   a. Beef – 24 to 48 hours

   b. Pork – 24 to 48 hours

   c. Poultry – 18 to 24 hours

    d. Fish – 4 to 8 hours

9. During the last 30 minutes of the suggested cooking time, add the fresh herbs (if you are using any).

10. Remove the pot from heat.

11. Let the contents cool down for about 30 minutes.

12. Strain out the bones, vegetables, and fat.

13. Transfer into your preferred container.

14. Consume immediately, or store in the freezer for later use. When frozen, the broth may last for 3 to 4 months.

Yield

Makes 20 to 24 servings

Congratulations! You have just completed the full kick-start plan for fasting. Your next step is to sustain the healthy eating habits that you have gained throughout the entire duration of this course.

Another example of a fasting plan and its advantages can be how to lose 10 pounds of quick fat. Have you ever had the difficulty of losing 10 pounds and eventually succeeded only to see it come back (plus more!) later? You probably wonder if any diet approach can work. Intermittent fasting plan is here to save the day.

It mainly involves alternating fasting periods with a food window. These times can be daily. For example, a fast 16 hours a day. Another option is to do a 24-hour fast once or twice a week. Both approaches work well and help to shed 10 pounds.

So what are the benefits of this type of food compared with other dietary plans? There are three main advantages:

To start with, it is easy to follow an intermittent fasting plan. You don't have to count calories, and at the right time, you don't have to worry about having to eat the right food. The duration of the speed/feed cycle can match your life.

Another benefit can be the fact that, you can eat until you are full. You can eat after fasting for most of the day without being limited and permanently hungry, a major dietary problem, and a significant reason for failure. As an additional bonus, most people adapt very quickly to the period they do not eat and are now mentally alert.

Also, it can easily be part of a long-term lifestyle choice instead of a short-term diet. This means that you probably had the end of the rebound weight gain many times before.

By now, you would also have a better idea of which fasting method works best for you. In case you have not noticed, each day of the kick-start plan represents different forms of fasting, as discussed in an earlier chapter of this book.

Refer back to your journal and check which days have felt good for you. Ask yourself why those days are different from the rest. Your answer would help you determine the right kind of fasting for you.

Chapter 10 – Examples of Simple and Light Gymnastics in Support of Fasting

To get the optimal results out of fasting, you must regularly exercise your body. You do not, however, have to go to the gym every day, or purchase expensive exercise equipment to meet this requirement. You should know how high the quality of your training routine is for your cardiovascular conditioning. Whether you are an athlete or a chronic exercise junkie, you need superior cardiovascular strength to endure the length of your training. Discover how the benefits of aerobic training high intensity will help you do this.

The advantages of high-intensity aerobic exercise like many forms of strength training, many types of cardiovascular fitness are also present. If you look at your workouts, you may structure your cardiovascular workouts to be either lower in intensity to last for more extended periods, or structure them to be high in power, so that your heart rate gets faster and more work in a shorter period. You can do circuit or even cross-training in your workout plan, including interval, for instance, to achieve a significant conditioning effect.

With a training program that dramatically increases your perceived level of exercise, you can raise your fitness in a far more profound way. It makes sense for me because you get your heart rate up quickly, and often you can adapt your nervous system much quicker. If you do this, you can make sure you are ready for most real events, whether you are training for a marathon or looking for a football match on the gridiron.

There's no doubt that you can cater more specifically to your training events. Still, for most athletes or fitness junkies, there is always room and a significant benefit for the incorporation of intermittent high strength cardio exercises into their training schemes. Even if you look at your strength plan, you can add a considerable conditioning function to it by controlling the time between sets and the frequency (lifted by weight) during your training. Do not always believe you can get your fitness from only "running" and "cycling." As the old saying goes, "There's more than one way to skin a cat."

If you ask about the benefits of high-intensity cardiovascular work, it must be assumed that the person seeking high-intensity cardiovascular workout is capable of doing so first. Remember that everything depends on continuous practice, so it makes no sense for a deconditioned person to exercise appropriately immediately if he or she doesn't even move first, which is the value of cardioversion with a lower intensity. When the deconditioned individual has progressed to an acceptable conditioning stage, the high-intensity exercise can be carried out often.

The time factor also has to be a massive advantage of high-intensity cardiovascular exercise. If you are one of these people who is always concerned of not having enough time to train or do a good workout, then you need a few exercising cardiovascular training books to visit. Even for athletes, there can be only little time to "do the job" and make sure they do not go low of their strength and conditioning objectives. High-intensity cardio-conditioning can be so valuable on fasting. This allows you to do a lot of work in a shorter period.

There are various easy and simple exercise programs that you can perform in the comforts of your home, and without the aid of complex gym tools. When carried out properly, these physical exercises can enhance the positive effects of fasting on your health by:

- speeding up the fat-burning process;
- fostering the development of muscles; and
- promoting the production of healthier cells.

The following are three simple and light gymnastics that are highly recommended for those going through a fasting program. Take note that these exercises do not require any gym equipment—just wear comfortable workout clothes and shoes, and you're all set.

For your guidance, the step-by-step routines for each exercise routine are also provided below.

A. Push-Ups

Many fitness experts consider the simple push-up as one of the best upper-body exercises, mainly due to the scope of its effects. Studies show that push-ups can build up the strength in the following areas of the body:

- Triceps
- Chest
- Shoulders
- Abdomen

Though it is commonly taught during gym class, most people still fail to observe the correct form for this exercise. To keep you from being one of them, here are the steps you need to follow to do a perfect push-up:

1. Lie down with your stomach and chest flat against the floor.

2. Keep each arm close to their corresponding side of your body.

3. Lift both arms in a backwards motion as high as you can while keeping your elbows straight.

4. Bend your elbows at a 90-degree angle.

5. Place your hands firmly on the floor.

6. Tuck in your toes together.

7. Stiffen your entire body as if you are a single plank of wood.

8. Push your body off the floor until your arms are straight and perpendicular to the floor.

9. Lower down your body to the floor while keeping your elbows tight.

You are doing this right if your chest, stomach, and hips are moving up and down together at the same rate. Otherwise, your body would move in wave-like fashion, which is not the proper form for a push-up.

How many push-ups should you do?

For most beginners, experts recommend doing only 15 repetitions per day. You may increase this number as you become more familiar and comfortable with the forms and motions involved in this exercise. Some people challenge themselves further by doing harder variations of the push-up, such as the one-arm push-up, and the one-leg push-up.

You may consider going beyond the standard push-up as well, but only if you are not ruthlessly forcing your body to do so. Try to keep your routines as simple and light as possible while you are still going through a fast.

B. Get-Ups

This is arguably the most comprehensive exercise routine that you can do without the aid of any special equipment. Designed to move every joint in your body, the Turkish get-up—or simply referred to as the get-up—would strengthen your shoulders, mid-section, and hips when done properly and regularly.

Learn how to do the get-up by following these steps:

1. Lie down on the floor on your back.

2. Extend out your arms and legs at a 45-degree angle away from your body—as if you are a starfish, or if

148

you are about to make a snow angel on the ground.

3. Press your right arm against the middle bone of your chest.

4. Lift and bend your right knee while keeping your right heel planted on the area of the floor that is close to your right buttock.

5. To initiate the roll up, push your right heel hard against the floor while extending up your right arm overhead.

   Tip: Imagine yourself holding up a cup of water in your right hand. Do not let the water spill out of the cup when you do the next steps.

6. Pull hard your left elbow against the floor to drive your chest up.

7. Keep yourself propped up using your left forearm.

8. Move your body upward from your right forearm to your right hand.

9. Keep your right arm extended up with your fists closed tightly.

10. Form a full bridge by driving your hips up with another push of your right heel on the floor.

11. Sweep your left leg back under your hips.

12. Position your left knees in an L-position with your left hand.

13. When you are ready, simultaneously lift up your left hand from the floor and rotate your right leg in order to adapt the overhead lunge position.

    Reminder: Your leg movement should look like the windshield wiper of a car. The back of your calf should swing in an outward manner until both of your knees are pointing at the same direction.

14. Straighten up from the lunge position while keeping your right arm extended up overhead.

15. Keep your gaze straight as you maintain this position for as long as you can comfortably do so.

16. Repeat the same steps with the other side of your body.

How many get-ups should you do?

Given that this is an extensive workout for your body, you should aim for only 2 sets of 3 repetitions for each side of your body per day. Do not use weights when doing this exercise until you have completely mastered each movement. Otherwise, you would end up with the wrong form, which would negate the positive effects of this routine on your body.

C. Squats

Since this exercise engages all the primary muscle groups in the lower region of your body, squatting can do wonders to the strength and form of your legs, thighs, and buttocks. However, like the push-up, many people do not know how to do a proper squat.

At the most basic level, squatting must be executed as if you are going to sit down on a chair. By doing so, you would have a higher chance of properly driving your hips back as you do a squat.

Keep this mindset while you follow these steps on performing a squat:

1. Move down your hips as deep as you can while keeping your thighs in a parallel position to the floor.

   Reminder: If you have an existing knee condition, avoid going beyond a 90-degree angle with your hips.

2. Stabilize your footing by firmly sticking your heels on the floor.

3. Keep your knees aligned with the tips of your toes.

4. As you squat, allow your torso to maintain its natural tilt.

   Reminder: A stiff and erect upper body would put more strain on your knees and would prevent your hips from being properly released from its current squatting position.

5. Return to an upright standing position by straightening your legs, but without moving your feet from their position on the floor.

How many squats should you do?

The optimal number of squats depend on whether or not you are using weights while doing this exercise. Since the instructions given above do not require any form of weights, you may aim for a safe target of 3 sets of 10 to 20 repetitions every other day.

You may do squats on a daily basis, in case you are wondering. However, the recommended schedule would give your body enough time to recover from the strain. Remember, your goal for performing squats is to enhance the effects of fasting on your health—not to build the muscles in your lower regions.

Fasting, by itself, can be beneficial to your body in various significant ways. So can exercising. Therefore, combining them in a balanced and proper manner would dramatically increase the benefits that you may expect from each activity.

You are free to explore other exercise routines that would fit best with your capabilities and schedule. Just remember to take the time in assessing your condition and progress periodically.

Chapter 11 - Detoxify with Water Fasting and Juice Fasting

Cleansing and detoxifying the skin is essential. The first thing I want to know when someone asks me about this matter is what they want to clean/disinfect precisely. Is there any other explanation? Maybe they are trying to lose weight, alcohol, heavy metals, to get away from drugs, to get rid of the metabolic waste, and caffeine. The purpose you purify defines the form you will have to use and quite often cleansing isn't necessarily to do to achieve a health goal. Maybe you aim to get more energy, and the reason you do not have any power is that you have a nutritional deficit or an endocrine imbalance. Before you choose a method, you need to know the reasons behind the symptoms.

Science shows that caloric limits have the benefits of optimal health and intermittent fasting to slow down aging biological processes. But it's hard to implement such techniques in a world full of calorie-rich, low nutrient foods and a society that insists on food every hour of the day.

We do not have to eat small mini-meals all day long, unlike common myths, to stabilize blood sugar, speed metabolism, and a slender physique. This day-long snack practice destroys your levels of blood sugar and insulin and allows them to rise and fall all day, even if you snack on "healthy" mini foods that contain a small amount of protein, fat, and fiber. Ideally, you want your insulin and blood sugar to rise as much as possible for a FEW times a day. This means eating only 2 or 3 meals a day, no snacks.

It is essential to reduce the frequency of eating between meals, when you consume snacks, to only 2 to 3 times a day before you go into the practice of intermittent fasting. It could take some days for your body to adjust to eating two or three times a day, during which you will experience symptoms of jittery, weakness, headaches, or nausea. This happens because you have trained your body to ask for a constant energy supply of food with eating a few mini-meals during the day instead of using glycogen stores in your liver and muscles (and eventually fatty acid storage from your fat cells) for energy. You cannot use your glucometers for energy because the constant supply of food calories gradually produces a lenient liver (and a sensation of weightlessness and heaviness), which is why it is vital to use glycogen energy regularly.

The most effective way to purify the liver is not to take special "liver cleansing" pills, to wash salts/olive oil, or to take laxatives or enemas. The best way of cleansing the liver by allowing it to deplete its glycogen storage is to use water for a short time quickly! Your liver will store between 250-500 calories in the form of glycogen depending on your body's size, to be used when all calories have been used up. Depending on your body size, your muscles will store 800-2000 calories as glycogen. These glycogen stores in your liver and muscles are used for energy before your body starts mobilizing stored fat for energy. Fasting on water for 24-48 hours once or every second week can increase energy levels, offer huge anti-aging benefits, improved sleep quality and enhance the performance of sports, safely rest your body from digestion and allow your liver and muscles to purify themselves and detoxify themselves.

Juice Fasting Another great way of relaxing, cleaning, and restoring the body is through healthy seasonal juice. Juice fasting rapidly enters the mainstream, as specific juice cleaning programs and raw food restaurants have made it easy for people who for some reason can't make a juice maybe because they are too short in time to make a fresh juice on a regular basis each day. One thing you should watch out for in the juice-based program is that they rely heavily upon high-glycemic fruit juices that are high in calories, fat, or fiber, including possible added sweeteners such as honey or agave when they are prepared at a shop. This has the opposite effect which is calorie depletion and a minimal impact on blood sugar. The diet of fruit juice can cause candida yeast to be overgrown in the digestive tract, causing systemic yeast and associated symptoms of health such as exhaustion, nausea, gaining weight, brain fog, skin problems, and persistent vaginal yeast infections.

If you're interested in preparing your seasonal juice, you can buy your juicer to save some money while preparing your own customized vegetable juice recipes. If you are not seriously ill, juice cleansing can be very safe and beneficial to your health for a period of 3 to 10 days. During this time, you should be able to do your usual daily activities, although additional rest and light exercise are recommended. ALWAYS listen to and respect what your body says, and, if you feel extreme pain in any fasting or cleansing program, don't do so until you have a medical specialist qualified in fasting supervision under direct medical control. Only in the residential fasting center can extended health fasting be performed.

Metabolism Boost

- 1 tablespoon of broccoli sprouts
- 1 tablespoon of laciniate
- 1 1/2 tablespoon of roman salad
- 1/3 of tablespoon of celery leaves
- 1 tablespoon of tomato
- 1/4 of a cup of red and yellow bell pepper
- 1 slice of cayenne pepper
- 2 tablespoon coconut oil
- 1 tablespoon MSM Crystals
- 1 raw egg

Instructions: Broccoli juice sprouts, kale, cucumber, sugar, tomatoes, bell pepper and cayenne pepper. In a food processor or mixer mix the juice with the coconut oil, cayenne pepper, MSM, raw egg. Get yourself to drink and feel the burn!

Morning Energizer

- 1/2 cup of roman lettuce
- 1/2 cup of coconut
- 1/2 cucumber• one beet
- five celery leaf
- 1/2 cup of ginger slice
- 1 tsp cocoa
- 1 tsp of cocoon
- 5-8 drops of a candida cleanse
- 1/2 cup of ginger

Take high-quality probiotics such as life colloids, which also contain zeolites and lithophilic earth minerals to reprogram hung mineral cells and boost detoxification of all your body's molds and mycotoxins.

Also, keep in mind that using a far-infrared sauna allows your body to release accumulated toxins from your body's tissues through your sweat. The water also increases your central body temperature, which boosts your basal metabolic rate to facilitate fat loss and a variety of diseases.

Fasting is an excellent way to detox, weight loss, and health improvements. Unfortunately, it is often difficult for most people living in our fast-growing society to spend time changing their habits and learn how to quickly. It's also a slightly intimidating operation. The 24-hour fasting is an easy way to get you going! This is a great way to try fasting. It's also perfect for your overall health. Let's talk about it in more detail.

Fasting is achieved in two primary ways: 1) Fasting water, and 2) Fasting concentrate. Water fasting is only recommended for professional fasters. Fasting juice is much more user-friendly and very effective. People can fast anywhere from one to thirty days, but some people go even longer. For most people, a fast 1-3 day is the best way to go, which will significantly benefit you. A new and effective quick way is known as intermittent speeding, in which people quickly spend several weeks 24-

48 hours once a week. Some even benefit from fasting a partial day, like a 12 hour fast overnight. The critical aspect of juice fasting is not to eat solid foods, only liquids. It gives your organism a rest from the digestion of solid food that takes a lot of energy. Fasting does three essential things.

1. It helps clean up your body's toxin system.
2. It may help relieve disease
3. kick your body into good health.

The juice is packed with vitamins and nutrients, especially organic and vegetable juices that are non-pasteurized. Green juices with fasting are highly recommended. The citrus extract can also be perfect for washing, in particular, lemon juice. Some use cranberry juice, another good cleanser. Juice contributes to the purification process and also provides you with energy and essential nutrients. The juice is easy to digest for the liver, making it ideal for fasting.

Chapter 12 - The No-Excuses Path to Weight Loss and Detox

After following any liquid diet, such as a juice, the way you break the fast is maybe more critical than the process. It is recommended to enter solid food program very slowly and use a digestive enzyme supplement during at least a couple of weeks after any prolonged juice fasting to prevent unpleasant reactions like bloating or fatigue after eating.

There is fasting and quickness, and stop eating isn't the way to lose weight quickly and correctly. To maintain a healthy metabolism and immune system, everyone needs a certain amount of food every day in their diets, and starving the body from any of the critical components in their biochemistry is going to risk your life in the name of weight loss.

Some celebrities claim that they have been on detox diets with only water and fiber to clear up their impurity system. The only scientific evidence there is that they have lost weight. How can we quickly lose weight?

It is very dangerous to go absolutely without food for reasons mentioned above. Your body has particular nutritional needs, particularly specific vitamins and herbal chemicals (phytochemicals) that help your immune system and metabolism. Therefore, the claim that we only eat liquid foods, and no solids can cause our body to burn fat does hold no truth. All the valuable components of our diet are lower water and fat-soluble liquids, and what causes the body to burn fat is not a lack of solid food, but a lack of carbohydrates in your diet. Nevertheless, you should be able to reduce weight and still eat enough nutrients to maintain the essential biochemical processes in your body by adding enough fruit and vegetable juices into your liquid diet and taking about three pints of purified water each day.

Preparing for such things quickly helps your body get the best advantage. Many claim that colon cleansing can help reduce the effects of any digestive problems, although it is controversial. It won't do any harm, though, so if you feel it can help you offer a psychological boost.

It is also important not to stuff yourself full of carbohydrates before fasting, as your weight loss is delayed or even prevented. This is not the way to quickly lose weight. It is vital that rapid weight loss also results in healthy weight loss, and food is neither healthy nor sensible before fasting.

This can damage your system unnecessarily by depriving your system of nutrition. Take into account your fasting reason-to lose weight. How quickly you lose weight properly is not focused on not eating food, but to force your body to use your fat deposit to feed your metabolism as a source of energy. You should be able to do so while maintaining a sufficient diet intake to avoid permanent or prolonged damage to your immune system or other bodily processes.

How can you move securely to accomplish that? Take your daily routine into account. You should not fast until you can stop doing a difficult job or be involved in dangerous situations when you feel weak. Fasting has effects with a few people when they find themselves in difficult situations, and also during menstruation, you shouldn't fast.

Decide whether you plan to fast for an extended period or only for two or three days at a time with interim eating periods. If latter, what should be your diet during periods of fasting? Some of them combine an occasional full fasting program with juice, but here again you have to be vigilant that your core processes is not put at risk. To remain functional, your liver needs a degree of nutrition.

If you're not used to fasting, it's harder to do without food for more than a day, but that's all you might need. Not only will you give your digestive system a well-earned rest, but also the foundation of a healthy weight loss plan that does not jeopardize your well-being. That's how to lose weight quickly.

This reduces the effect of prolonged fasting on your body two to three times per month and helps to remove many of the toxins in your system. When you break quickly, take two glasses of salted lemon water to flush the system, and then have a regular breakfast.

By incorporating this into a healthy approach to weight loss, you feel better about yourself and will be more likely to permanently lose weight and will increase your metabolism, which will help you to lose weight more quickly.

Intermittent fasting has always been a popular way to use the natural fat burning capacity of your body to lose fat in a short time. But many people want to know, if sporadic fasting works, and how does it work precisely? If you do not eat for an extended period, your body changes the way it processes hormones and enzymes, which can help you lose weight. These are the key advantages and how we accomplish here gains.

Metabolic functions include the speed at which you burn fat and is dependent on hormones. Your body produces the growth hormone and encourages fat breakdown in the body to provide energy. When you rapidly increase the body's growth, hormone production does too for a while. Fasting also reduces the amount of insulin in the bloodstream to ensure the body burns fat instead of storing it.

A short time of fasting which lasts 12-72 hours increases the level of metabolism activity and adrenaline, which increases the number of calories that you consume. People who quickly gain energy through increased adrenaline also do not feel tired even if they don't collect calories in particular. While you think that fasting will lead to lower fuel, the body compensates for this by maintaining a high calorie burning regime.

Some people eat sugar instead of fat every 3-5 hours. Fasting will change the metabolism of burning fat for more extended periods. At the end of a 24-hour fast day, your body has spent around 18 hours burning through the body's fat stores. Intermittent fasting can help to increase fat loss for anyone who is regularly active but still struggles with fat loss without the need for a dramatic dietary plan alteration.

Another advantage of intermittent fasting is that it resets the body of a person. Going for a day without eating changes the appetite of a person and makes him or her feel hungry over time. When you struggle with food, intermittent fasting will help your body adapt to periods when you do not eat and help you not always feel hungry. Many people are noticing that they start to eat healthier and be more in control of their diet.

Intermittent fasting varies but is typically prescribed every week for around one day. An individual may have a fluid, nutrient-filled smoothie or another low-calorie alternative during this day. As the body adapts to an irregular period of fasting, this usually is not necessary. Intermittent fasting tends to gradually reduce fat stores through a metabolism that breaks up fat rather than sugar or muscle. It has been successfully used by many people and is an easy way to make a positive change. Intermittent fasting provides a simple, effective option for fat loss and a healthy lifestyle to anyone tired of the traditional diet.

Enough is enough. Enough is enough. It's NOW the time to lose weight and clean up my dear friend. Life is too short. Life is too short. Let us not allow any valuable time to go to waste with obesity and diseases.

Why not seek to fast intermittently? Some people think that if they don't fast for days and days, they can't achieve their goals. That's not the case. However, fasting can be just as effective intermittently. It can give you incredible health benefits; both in body and in spirit. Any time the digestive system can relax and concentrate on purification would help.

If your boss says, "you can go home for that day." Do you refuse because he doesn't give you all the week off? Or are you going to jump for a few hours to rest? Of course! Of course! You'd go home, okay? Well, the digestive system is like that. It is very grateful for the rest, even though you only stop eating for a few hours.

This is at the very heart of what is all about intermittent fasting.

Intermittent fasting means you choose those hours and days that you do not consume solid food. You can instead drink water or juice, depending on the type of pace you want to do. Fasting with water will only increase the loss of weight, but also make it harder.

As a beginner, start fasting with a drink. Better to lower the fruit in it. In other words, make yourself convenient. If you wish, you can always go for more extended periods later. Remember always: slow is fast. It's not a race.

This is why intermittent fasting is so good. Maybe not everyone can fast 30 days, but almost everyone can skip a meal several times a week or fast for a 24-hour cycle. Whether you have fasted successfully in the past or not this type of plan will work for you. This wipes away any doubts and reasons for not taking action. Let's look at several intermittent fasting strategies you may take into account.

The slowest way to go is to skip a meal three days a week... Lunch generally. Eat your breakfast as usual when you wake up. You can then quickly go through lunch and finish with a responsive dinner by evening. This is similar to the fast form some do in the lent season. We fast every day from sunset to sunset for 40 days.

Another option is to fast for 24 hours (for example from 8 a.m. to 8 a.m.) and then eat normal (but healthy) for 24 hours. You can run "every other day." Most people do so indefinitely before they meet their weight loss and wellness objectives.

Let's go a little further. You can also fast half a week, i.e., breakfast Monday morning and promptly through Thursday night. How's that sound? You break soon with a small salad, steamed veggies, or fruit.

Every week intermittent fasting is a bit harder but very powerful. In other words, from Sunday to Sunday, you probably revert to eating and then fasting again for the same amount of days. So you would fast for a whole seven days "every other week."

And what will you do? It is better to skip one meal every few days than to do nothing. The 1000-kilometer journey begins with the first move.

Or maybe you're afraid to fast. There are many misunderstandings about this discipline. Many people can tell you that if you don't feed every day, you'll "die." Or that the body fails because of lack of nutrition. Nevertheless, fasting does not deteriorate health in most situations. Alternatively, it strengthens!

In the end, you're not alone. Many adopt this incredible discipline and see remarkable results. Think about your motives. Why do you want to fast? What do you think you're going to gain from that? Cementing your goals and motivation will help you achieve this.

Consider this "day" your choice to start to achieve your goals for your health and weight loss. There are no reasons for not prioritizing this. What is more important than your wellbeing?

What's going to happen to your loved ones if you get ill? Which price are you willing to pay for NOT taking action in your mind and body? Any hunger or pain we experience when fasting is little compared to the HUGE benefits we earn for our wellbeing. You can see your life continually changing. You can do that.

There are many intermittent fasting benefits to improve your life that are found by scientists who have to limit caloric intake for one reason or another. There are several periodic fasting benefits. Intermittent fasting is defined as not eating approximately 15 hours. Many features of the body can be changed with this technique. The real question is not whether fasting can or shouldn't help you, but how it can and shouldn't help you.

Fasting has shown that blood pressure is lower, and HDL levels are higher. It can help you manage diabetes considerably and also helps you lose weight. All these sound quite good and this type of fasting can be achieved. Studies conducted on various animal species indicate that reducing caloric intake increases their lives by up to 30 percent.

Human studies show that blood pressure, blood sugar, and insulin sensitivity are increasing. With these tests, it is reasonable that fasting for a more extended period increases the life of human beings. The same results can be achieved by cutting your calories by 30% every time, but depression and irritability have been shown in these cases. Fasting is a remedy that is provided instead of simply cutting calories and has benefits without stress or irritability.

Intermittent fasting works when you eat food every other day. On the days you eat, you will finally be able to consume almost twice as much food as you would normally. You will still get the same quality of calories, but you have all the advantages. It reduces stress levels and improves your overall health. This form of fasting is an ideal way to enhance your physical condition, live a longer life, and always feel better.

It's certainly no surprise to you that a number of diets and exercise regimes were credited for weight loss. Many of them, perhaps most, are perfectly valid. Some of them are complete scams and others just aren't very effective. Any program that claims that it is too good to be true does not deserve your time. Some of the most popular and effective approaches are discussed here.

Most people will lose any weight if they eat fewer calories or more than normal. However, they often reach a plateau where there is no more weight loss or a slow loss. This is not a problem for those who only have a few pounds to lose. But it may not be enough for those who have much to lose.

The quality of the food is also significant. Many people find that they simply lose peso while eating less calories by improving their diets, replacing fast foods with, high-quality, fruits fresher vegetables, and lean protein. The difference is that in fresh, whole foods the nutritional value provides more of what the body needs, so that they are used instead of stored as fat. People are getting more energy and more active rather than being slowed down by low-quality food.

This is the most successful approach to weight loss. It is the best way to continue to lose weight and develop lifelong habits that help to maintain weight. A lack of activity, not over-alimentation, is the main cause of overweight for most people.

However, as mentioned above, the quality of food consumed must be considered. You may not actually have to reduce calories, but you should be sure you eat healthy foods. Know about food and make intelligent decisions.

Training is important, so you mostly lose fat and keep most of your muscle. If you are not exercising, you lose both, leading to a flabby appearance of "skinny fat" not to mention the harm to your health in general. Weightlifting and cardio exercise should be performed by those who try to lose weight.

This method has been made very famous recently among both professional and novice athletes who want to lose weight. This looks very effective and is much healthier than fasting or low-calorie diets. In fact, several significant health benefits have been shown.

The rule of intermittent fasting is that you eat one large meal quickly for the rest of the day, rather than eating your meals at various times throughout the day.

Research has shown that this way of eating enhances insulin sensitivity and mitochondrial power that leads to better disease control and slows down signs of aging. The decreased oxidative stress makes every cell in the body strong and resilient. Such findings shocked scientists as they expected to find a long period of fasting detrimental to health.

The best time to feed is two hours is in the evening. This is true because energy is redirected from your nervous system if the parasympathetic nervous system is triggered. For this reason, you sometimes feel sleepy after a big meal: your body is designed to rest while your nutrients are being assimilated. Make the most of it and have your lunch if you can do so without upsetting your schedule.

Make sure during your two-hour feeding time you obtain enough calories. Especially at the beginning, this can be difficult. Men should eat at least 1800 calories per day, and women should eat at least 1200 calories per day. Don't violate the principle that healthy foods are eaten simply to get calories, because you are short of nutrients.

It's all right to have water and tea during your fasting period and you can even have a small number of green vegetables or berries. The foods are digested so easily that they do not counteract the advantages of quick food.

The best solution is to plan your exercise with a small, protein-rich meal, 15 to 30 minutes before you go to work out, followed by a bigger meal afterwards, during your feeding period.

Many types of procedures are done to induce weight loss. Only people who are clinically obese (100 pounds for men and 80 pounds for women overweight) are eligible for surgery, and other health issues may affect eligibility. Surgery is a last resort, but it was the remedy that many people had reached that stage.

Such surgical procedures reduce the amount of food you can take and eat. Lap-band activity requires the implantation of a system that limits the ability of the abdomen to expand. Other methods remove the entire portion of the stomach or insert a space-saving balloon.

The intestinal resection recirculates the intestines so that calories are less consumed. Those who have undergone such surgery cannot also absorb as many nutrients, so supplements are typically required.

Operation is risky, but can be successful. Those who were unable to lose weight by conventional methods not only enjoyed weight loss, but other benefits such as diabetes reversal, reduced risk of stroke and heart attack and increased lifespan.

You should adhere to changes in lifestyle including healthier meals and physical exercise in order to lose weight. It has been said that it takes 28 days to develop a new habit, so give yourself a month and you will probably enjoy feeling healthy, energetic and strong.

It takes dedication to succeed, but don't feel like a failure if you slip down the road. No one's perfect, so take a break.

You may find another way to lose weight quickly, but it would require that you are more physically active. Nevertheless, a much more formal training plan, in addition to simple daily physical activity, may be appropriate for women who want to boost their health or who want to lose weight. Your program should cover the four fitness components, including one aerobic activity, continuous activity with all your body muscles, enhance cardiovascular conditioning, and decrease additional fat. Walking, jogging, biking, swimming, and aerobics, or training courses and videos are all aerobic activities.

You do it too soon, and you can get hurt, exhausted, and discouraged. Experts suggest seasoned exercisers with 60 minutes per session and do not exceed 200 minutes of aerobic fitness exercise per week.

Strength training, for example, by raising a weight, improves muscle strength and persistence, increases metabolism, helps maintain bone density, and causing more calories to burn.

Extensive exercises, quick, gentle movements that stretch the muscles, including fast, enhance flexibility. Such actions are often performed in workouts or videos and are also part of yoga.

But how much is sufficient? One of the most common questions is,' how much do I need to practice?' Centers for Disease Control and Prevention in the United State and other professional groups advise healthy women to conduct some aerobic exercise for 30 to 45 minutes on most or all days of the week. Such minutes will accumulate— 15 minutes in the morning of an aerobic video and 15 minutes in the evening, for example. Intermittent exercise can be part of an efficient weight-loss strategy because, after every workout, your metabolism is increased. If you are inactive, you will have to get to work slowly. Start every second day with five or ten minutes or anything you are comfortable with, and add every other session for one minute.

Similarly, training in resistance should not be overlooked. Facilitate yourself, with lighter weights, and later get to more weights and repetitions. You don't need to practice much more than three days a week and try to wait no less than 48 hours for the same muscle group to provide the muscles with enough time and energy to heal between the workouts.

Extension and mobility should be achieved for 10 to 12 minutes for three times during a period of seven days. Three times - seven days. You may attend a training session. You can even make lighter stretches of your desk. Stretching degrees include shoulder and leg circles. Various areas are mainly concentrated on the muscles of the neck, back, chest, thigh, and leg.

Your second question is, "How hard can I practice?" You must also increase the intensity of the exercise while you work on improving the duration of your training. Low-intensity workouts, such as homework, gardening, and dog walking provides significant benefits to your fitness but, especially when weight loss is one of your objectives, in order to seriously improve fitness, you need to increase your ante and work with moderate or higher intensity with vigorous activities individual tennis, including fast walking or jogging, aerobics or cycling.

In reality, women who are trying to lose weight will benefit from moderate intensity exercise at most, as you will need endurance practice. The 201 exercise duration and intensity trial included overweight, healthy women between 21 and 45 years. All received reduced-calorie meals and were allocated physical activity schemes 1 out of 4 years old. The routine also involves moderate to intense exercises for a shorter duration (2.5 to 3.5 hours weekly) and longer (3.5 to 5 hours weekly). The physical activity was primarily a fast walk, and about 900 to 1000 calories were used daily in regimes.

Women lost a vital weight level to all four groups— about 13 to 20 pounds (8 percent— 10 percent) and kept their weight loss for every year. Their calories have enhanced their spiritual health. But most significantly, in the list of four groups, how much weight loss and fitness improvement was the same. The writer concluded that an intervention program would initially promote the adoption and maintenance of moderate-intensity training with a minimum of 150 minutes each week, if possible, and, ultimately, the transition towards a workout level of 60 minutes every day, most days of the week. This higher level complies with the recommendation of the Institute of Medicines, for children and adults published in the 2002 Dietary Reference Intakes Report, of 60 minutes each day, regardless of weight.

Since the fitness goal is to work your heart muscle, the workout will boost your heartbeat. One way to determine whether you exercise intensively is to test the heart rate. Your heart rate should be approximately 70 to 85% of the limit. The average heartbeat for the start minute is 220. Take your pulse after about five minutes of warming up and aerobic activity, and place two fingers around the radial artery on your wrist. Count beats for approximately 10 secs.

Chapter 13 – Final Words

Above all else, what would you like to do? What do you hate? How would your life be different if you could always do what you want and never worry about doing the things you loathe? Perhaps, quite good, right? Yes... and... No. Yes.

Come on. Come on. Let's take a second to think about it. What if life was all butterflies and rainbows—and you never had obligations? You may not believe me, but it's true. When you stop and ponder it for a second, it can happen.

Avoiding extra stress and doing things fast and efficiently (especially the less-than-pleasant something) is never wrong. It not only leaves more time for you to do just what you want, but it also makes you more comfortable—eventually leading to greater happiness. It is a significant thing to remember when you are inspired to be successful and to make things: the less you do what you hate, the more often you can do what you enjoy.

However, work sucks, right? Sure. Sure. It can. It can. If you're getting stuck, it can be awful whether it's the "necessary evil" stuff involved in working, sustaining a company and staying in shape–or "part of life" stuff like trying to maintain friendships and work on extra tasks, job–and life.

So don't get stuck down. Left. Right. Don't ever bust your ass, try to be lazy as often as you can, and try to avoid work, right? Not quite... Not quite...

Not that sipping mojitos on the beach is wrong if it's your thing for the rest of your days. It's only this: you have to realize that what you want to do, whether it's a whole lot of nothing, or anything-will always be a by-product of things you have to do effectively and quickly.

Here's a side note:

Assume it's something you don't want to do regardless of what your working version is. In reality, you are very likely to hate it. But since most people do the opposite in their free time, there is a good chance (unless they are fortunate) that hating or at least not being able to enjoy these responsibilities optimally, is probably the norm. But the point-and this needs to be underlined again - is that doing something you hate (or don't like i.e. responsibilities) would improve your ability to make whatever hell you do if there was nothing in your way.

So if you are lazy or vegetating out, then have it. Just realize that the fact is that intermittent effort will help you do what is needed and allow you to use more time doing what you love.

1. Figure out what is most important in your life—this is the essential step in getting things done since each next step depends on this. You need to determine what's most essential and where your priorities are (and straighten things out if they're wrong). If you know what is most important, a hierarchy of tasks can then be created based on its importance. Tackle the things that matter most and those that need to be completed before anything else can be accomplished.

2. Plan your tasks—the next step is to see what items should (or must) be achieved together once you've built a hierarchy to help with task importance. It applies to things that can be done together because you have the time or

liberty over a certain period to do things that should be done together merely out of convenience.

3. Use the Pareto principle-the Pareto principle is relevant for many realms of life, but when it comes to productivity, it is essential. If you do not know the Pareto (or even if you are and may be able to use a reminder) principle, this is the deal. It's the same as 80/20, and it means (for our purposes) that 20% of your effort produces 80% of your results. You could also argue that 20% of your overall efforts constitute an essential part of your job. Thought about it like this: most of the results come from a few attempts. If you can do most of your things, the rest is usually a breeze.

4. Use the Theory of Parkinson-this one is enormous. Parkinson's Law is the idea of expanding work to fill the time it has to be completed. That may sound somewhat esoteric or even supernatural at first, but the truth is rock solid. It's not mercurial, and it grows and shrinks completely alone. If we talk about the purpose of your life or simply what you want to do on a specific day, you are the master of your destiny. So the work doesn't expand to fill time. You stretch your work when you fail to set deadlines.

Get it now? Get it now? And, frankly, how true is that? If you don't set an expiration date, your tempo gets slower, your concentration is less focused, and your energy fluctuates like the flood. Let's explain one thing: you don't want your inspiration to be there for one minute and later vanish! While some mistakes are natural (and inevitable), when it is necessary, you need simple, focused motivation and power. The good thing about Parkinson's Law is that by design, you can maximize productivity because you set the right pace of work. Too soon to arrange your deadlines? The work is done (or not), but performance is affected.

Another mistake you may do is work over the smallest details and lose sight of your ultimate goal, or you will be lazy and never complete what you need to do. This is why you need to tinker somewhat with the deadlines, but while you set a target date or time that will give you the time you need to finish your stuff, you're good to go. You'll do more in less time while you'll get less (or nothing) without Parkinson's Law, and time spent is meaningless.

5. Trivialize the Unimportant-at first, it might sound like a misnomer, but here's the jus:

trivializing the unimportant sounds prominent and logically easy, but it may not be. Actually. Do it! Do it! It is incredibly powerful to break away from the crap in your life, close your ears to the noise, and focus on the few crucial things. Many people even know why it is perfectly useful. The problem is that most people are too distracted and unorganized to do so. But this is the cool part: you do not have to be highly organized and ultra-disciplined to make the first spring of discovery. Yes, it's good to try and be structured and disciplined, too, but if you're missing either, the goal isn't to try changing the whole individual overnight.

The best way to start trivializing the meaningless is to find out what is essential. Once you have figured out this, you must classify all these items as your 5%. So ask yourself, do these things make up the top five percent of your life? If they do, great. And if you have placed things that don't matter in that category, get rid of them. By the same token, if you left out some essential things, add them. The goal is to reduce your focus on the critical elements in your life. The remainder (yes, the other 95%) is not so important and was likely a pleasant emotional and physical space in your life. The key is to focus on the critical 5% and ignore the insignificant 95% because the majority of things in life are just that-trivial.

6. Visualize achievement–this is an unbelievably powerful strategy for doing things, and is often overlooked. Most people have heard of the display, but either they don't think it works or doesn't commit to shooting it. A lot of studies show that visualization can be used effectively for all things, from combating disease to improving prospects and productivity. The problem with people and their lack of results is that they seldom conform to this practice-if they try. But here's the thing– it doesn't take long to visualize, and it doesn't take a ton of time.

Not need to make a lot of effort. You don't have to do much when it comes to visualizing things that need to be done. The most effective strategy I have found is to see the goal or task as already finished. Well, meditate on the idea that whatever you try to do is already done. It sounds simple, but it's incredibly difficult. That's why: many people who have something to do, they don't even like to talk about the process. (side note: you have to be sure that you are unable to do something because it is not incongruous with your long-term goals or moral code) If you just like the idea of doing something just because you think it's going to be complicated or time-consuming, this form of visualization is for you, and you should be excited.

Once you have the idea that your goal is done in your mind-and, have already considered the task or goal to be completed-you will be much more likely to do it in reality. The reason is twofold: first, you will be more motivated and less concerned about the sequential steps involved. Secondly, you almost believed that the thing was already done. This means you'll do it unless you have a lot of inner conflict or frustration.

7. Do little every day–this may appear to be another little tip, but it's incredibly efficient and easy to follow. Whether we're talking about sorting your workplace, doing work, or doing things at work, it's imperative to pack yourself. Something has to be done right away. We get stressed because whatever we try is not done (and yesterday we wanted to do it). This is where it is essential to let go of your white knuckle grip to make a list. Be aware that while a time limit is reasonable, you must set a realistic time frame to get your stuff done. Then divide your task into smaller pieces and do it a little every day. Give yourself time and keep in mind that it's probably better to give yourself a little longer to do anything than hurry if this means that quality is compromised.

It doesn't have to be challenging to get things done, no matter what you're trying to do. When you set your goals from the start, you will be on the right track when you pace yourself, performance, and avoid distractions. Determine what you need for the next five, 11, and even 21 years and split the dream into its pieces. Figure out what steps to take, turn off the noise in your life, and start.

The increase in fasting for weight loss has recently been unbelievable. This is partly due to the flexibility and convenience that traditional diets do not work! Many of the old weight loss stigmas are slowly but surely disproved by research. Some of these old beliefs include things like' you have to eat every 2 hours to lose well,' and' your body will enter hunger mode unless your metabolism gets ticked.' If you just learned about intermittent fasting, you might wonder what it's all about.

Fasting is a state-of-the-art fat loss system used for weight loss as long as records reveal. Fortunately, our evolution meant that our bodies could store energy as fat when we eat a calorie excess and burn the same energy supplies when we run a calorie deficit! When we fast (even just under 16 hours) for a short time, we put our bodies in a calorie deficit, and when we have a calorie deficit, we burn fat! To lose as much fat as possible, a sensible nutritional plan is strongly recommended if you don't fast; you can include favorite foods provided they are moderate.

It might be even more straightforward than many of us assume to adapt to this new fasting way of life. Our hunger hormone Grehlin is inhibited when we fly. Many people are skeptical about attempting fasting, but the overwhelming majority of them are shocked after a fasting plan, such as Eat Stop Hunger.

It may not be practical for many people to eat every 2 hours or to exclude all foods, as is the case in many traditional diets. There are many solutions to intermittent fasting, including but not limited to Eat Stop Eat, The Warrior Diet, and the Leangains Method of Martin Berkhan. For example, Eat Stop Eat opts 24 hours quickly, once or twice a week, to place you in a safe calorie deficit. You eat with this approach every day! Brad Pilon, the author of Eat Stop Eat, suggests that one evening, you could stop eating 6 pm, and the following evening begins eating again at 6 pm!

The big thing about fasting is that you cannot lose fat all the time; you can do 20 hours instead of 24 hours. The versatility is great because you create the rules and are still tremendously beneficial.

The surprising thing about fasting is that your focus will dramatically increase, particularly during fasting. This is due to hormone releases when we fast, which allows us to focus our attention on important tasks and not on food! The mental clarity that you get from fasting is unbelievable; you get much more productive.

Your productivity will probably increase when you try to fast. You can focus on anything you like (not eating); anything you want, like reading, walking, writing, and working, will now receive your full attention! You may not believe that you'd always think about food, but try it a couple of times and see how efficient it can be.

Now let's talk 24 hours fasting! Here are my instructions-

1.   Hours of fast–dinner is most appropriate around 6 pm. Why? Okay, most of the time when you are sleeping and your body rests, you don't think about food. It seems to flow well with most people. Anytime is all right, but depending on your timetable.

2.   A few hours before fasting-eat lightly. Before fasting. Don't do solid and heavy food stuffing for yourself. Only eat light and healthy foods.

3.   Drinking Tea-Drink plenty of tea. Like green juice and carrot/beet not-pasteurized, but every vegetable combination is excellent. At least buy organic/natural non-filtered juice in cases where it is challenging to find non-

pasteurized juice. Lemon juice with water is another unique way to help cleanse the body (this is the basis of the 10-day Master's effective cleanse). And some people use Cranberry juice again, but it must be pure juice, not sugar or concentrate. Every juice is good, but only organic, natural, and only pure juice and water are not expected to be any other ingredients.

4.   Drink Cleansing Tea-Herbal & Green Tea will help your body cleanse. There are detox teas, and several fasting, Yogi Tea and traditional medicine are my favorites, or you can make your own. Teas and herbs are available in most natural or online food stores. Herbs are an essential way to help clean and fast. Drink a couple of cups in your fast.

5.   Drink Water-Water can purify and flush contaminants out. Drink lots of filtered water, including juice and tea, of course. For cleanliness and overall health, pure filtered water is vital.

6.   Eliminate toxins-urinate and bowel as much as possible. You often urinate while you drink fluids. Tea and raw juice, especially vegetable juices, will assist you in the elimination and purification of solid waste. Take a mild herbal tea laxative before, during, or right after washing if you need any assistance with bowel movements. The majority of laxative teas take a couple of hours

to work to help with a reliable removal. Many of the cleaning & detox teas are also helpful.

7.	Have a quiet time –meditate, pray, or have a quiet time to think. Concentrate on your body and feel quickly.

8.	Exercise-Get sweat; expel toxins from the skin pores. Make your body shift at least once or twice during your fast.

9.	After the fast-again, eat a few hours lightly. Don't eat a great meal. Eat healthily. Eat healthily. Lightly steamed veggies, no abundant proteins, are good, little portions. When you finish fasting at 6 pm, you can eat lightly, drink tea and go to bed and feel somewhat exhausted and refreshed. Another 8 hours of sleep cleaning will help.

The 24-hour fasting is an excellent way to try this program. It's long enough to do you well, but quick enough to do it without too much effort. Yeah, you may be hungry or without energy, but drink lots of fruit, tea, and coffee, and you're going to be okay. If you like the 24 hours fast, try a few weeks later 48 or 72 hours fast. Or work 24 hours quickly once a week or even once a month. It can be very beneficial for you to give your body rest even 24 hours a month with a fast one.

Conclusion

Is it safe to fast?

When it comes to weight loss, it is the method, in recent years, that has been much more widely used. Fasting is not a new idea, and it's probably one of the oldest weight control methods, actually quite the contrary, but that's a whole different story.

Whether or not fasting is safe is the issue which the medical and nutritional experts have raised several times, more often than not, although both are beginning to be much more open-minded on this often-controversial method of weight loss.

So... Is quicking safe?

Fasting generally involves food, liquids, or both, and self-deprivation. Again, fasting can occur in various kinds, such as fasting of fruits, intermittent, only water, or vegetable juice, etc. In many cases, though, people will abstain entirely from food intake. Unfortunately, the answer to the question when it comes to achieving objectives of rapid weight loss... Fasting is secure, not as cut and dry as many would hope since the answer is yes and no!

Moderation is suitable for most things, and fasting is no different. If you fast for too long, the effects can be harmful and lead to diseases ranging from anorexia to liver failure. Still, fasting can provide many advantages regularly, including a colonic and clearer skin as well as a weight loss.

While it is 100% true that the numerous types of fasts help people to lose weight quickly, it can also be true that a lot of this weight is fluid and not fat, well at least at first and only if you were at full swing, when you don't eat water, or food, by the way!

The reasons why weight loss should not take fasting into account and why it ought to be! Confused?

1. Fasting is slowing down your metabolism. This means that the fat you try to lose begins to burn at a much slower rate, so you stop losing weight. This is true, but what is not emphasized is how long you need to be in a rapid state to slow down your metabolism.

Look at it this way, everyone else is on a diet or two, but what all foods do, is to reduce the daily calorie intake. What we find out with all diets is that they all reach a plateau of weight loss, most of them around the first two weeks. A plateau is when the weight loss process of the previous two weeks either slows down significantly or stops entirely.

The reason for this is that the metabolism of the body has adapted to the new low-calorie intake, and once done, it will stop the fat reserves from being burned. Fasting will have the same effect for a long time and will reach a plateau too. However, intermittent 24-hour fasting periods won't influence your metabolism but will STILL reduce your weekly calorific consumption.

2. Fasting is not recommended for people with health problems. If someone has a health disorder or is taking drugs, fasting should be avoided, since it can quickly worsen such problems or weaken the immune system of the person. A balanced person needs all the nutrients he can get, while every person who uses certain medications requires substantial digestive material to safely ingest and even to help them work out their intended actions.

Most are right, but many medical conditions would greatly benefit from intermittent fasting, and there are alternative medications for most complaints that work without food. Remember, we're thinking about irregular fasting periods not approaching 24 hours, a quarter of which would be used to bed! I'm sure there are millions of Muslims and people from other religions that often take medicines safely and fast at the same time, for religious reasons. The safest option is to consult your doctor at all times.

Mostly, if fasting is safe depends entirely on the circumstances. If overlooked, it could pose a real danger to your wellbeing. Still, the path towards a healthy and natural weight loss is open if nutritional experts follow a sensible, easy guideline centered on scientifically proven ways.

First and foremost, hunger is unintentional abstinence from outside forces; it happens when food is scarce in times of famine and war. On the other hand, fasting is voluntary, deliberate, and monitored. Food is readily available, but we do not eat it for spiritual reasons, health reasons, or for other purposes.

Fasting does not have a regular duration. It can be done for a couple of hours to several days or months. Intermittent fasting is a mode of eating in which we cycle between fasting and regular food. In general, shorter 16-20-hour fasting is more frequent even daily. Longer fasts are done 2-3 times per week, usually 24-36 hours. As it happens, between dinner and breakfast, we all quickly spend about 12 hours each day.

Millions and millions of people have been fasting for thousands of years. Is it healthy? Is it healthy? No. No. Many studies have shown that it has enormous health benefits.

I'd like to thank you and congratulate you for transiting my lines from start to finish.

I hope this book was able to help you to discover the right fasting method for you.

The next step is to apply what you have learned from this book by creating a fasting plan that would work with your current lifestyle and help you achieve your personal fitness goals.

You should also go for a consultation with your physician as well in order to get their opinion about your plan to fast. Make sure that you would be able to fully commit to fasting once you have begun. Though the planning stage may take a long time, you should push through until you are completely certain about the details pertaining to this life-changing decision.

I wish you the best of luck!

RACHELE PARKESSON

Made in the USA
Middletown, DE
28 December 2019